AF871159

THE BACK PAIN SOLUTION

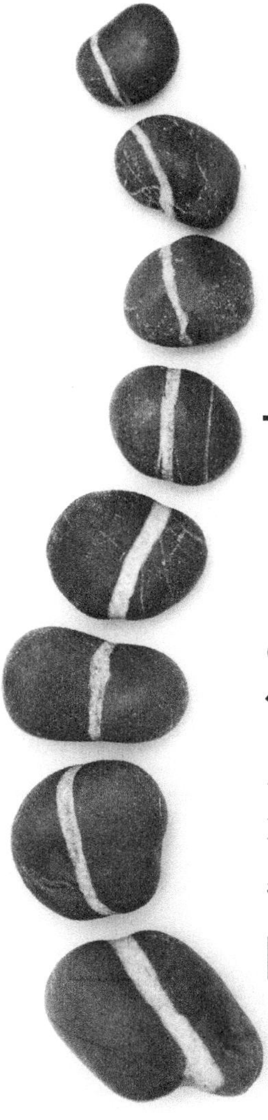

The Back Pain Solution

A Patient's Guide to Laser Spine Surgery, Minimally Invasive Procedures, and Avoiding Surgery Altogether

Michael Hasz, MD, FACS

LIONCREST
PUBLISHING

COPYRIGHT © 2021 MICHAEL HASZ

All rights reserved.

THE BACK PAIN SOLUTION

A Patient's Guide to Laser Spine Surgery, Minimally Invasive Procedures, and Avoiding Surgery Altogether

ISBN 978-1-5445-0839-9 *Paperback*

978-1-5445-0838-2 *Ebook*

Contents

Disclaimer: This book contains information as to the advances in medical health care and operative and non-operative treatment of various spinal conditions. It should be considered a reference but not a medical manual. Treatment should be individualized and focused, based upon specific diagnoses of an individual. If you know or suspect that you have a medical problem, you should seek competent medical and/or surgical care for your individual evaluation and treatment. The publisher and author disclaim any liability for outcomes which may occur after applying any of the treatments or procedures described in this book. There are never any guarantees in medicine, however, with advances in nutrition, health, exercise, non-operative, and operative care, many people will be able to improve their lives significantly and lead very productive, useful lives.

Introduction

When I was a young surgeon in training, spine surgery was undergoing a paradigm shift. I just didn't know it at the time. The days when back surgery involved putting you in a body cast for weeks or even months at a time were being put behind us. As an Air Force orthopedic surgeon at Andrews Air Force Base back then, we were just starting to use high-tech imaging and surgery that was far less invasive—and we could see how much better the results were for our patients.

Today, our diagnostic capabilities have improved. Technology such as an MRI lets us visualize the spine in amazing detail. At the same time, surgical treatment options have dramatically improved. We can now treat spine problems with better, safer methods using very small incisions that heal quickly. The latest developments in stem cell and other nonoperative treatments are being shown to work and are increasingly available to patients. The future will bring even more improvements, such as remote robotic surgeries performed by surgeons who could be anywhere in the world.

The treatment of spine problems today with nonsurgical options has become so effective that 80 to 90 percent of the patients I see don't need surgery at all. I can fix their back problems holistically, using nutrition, weight loss, physical therapy, exercise, and other lifestyle changes.

WHERE WE ARE TODAY

For decades, spine surgery was big surgery. To reach the spine, we had to make large incisions. After the surgery, some patients were immobilized for weeks in plaster casts that went from their knees to their chest. Complications such as blood clots were common; the immobilization meant tremendous loss of muscle tone and a long recovery period. Even worse, quite frequently, the surgery was not very helpful.

The development of minimally invasive surgery (MIS) changed all that. We now have ways to operate using microscopes and tiny instruments that are inserted through much smaller incisions—incisions so small that they may not even need stitches to close them. Other developments, such as artificial discs, bone cages, titanium screws, and other implants have shortened recovery times dramatically. Lasers let us treat many spine conditions without cutting through muscles and ligaments, leading to even smaller incisions and even faster recovery. Today, many of my surgical patients are up and walking almost as soon as they're awake. They usually go home the same day or after just a night or two in the hospital. Immobilizing casts are almost unheard of now.

Spine problems can now be diagnosed quickly and very accurately. X-rays, which have been around for well over a century, are still an important tool for imaging the spine, but we also use much more precise methods. The CT scan, which is just a more sophisticated X-ray, gives us a more detailed look at the spine. MRI scans provide amazingly detailed images, particularly of the nerves, discs, and other soft tissues. We use DEXA scans to detect osteoporosis and use diagnostic injections to see disc problems or find other causes of pain. SPECT scans can find microfractures of the vertebrae. We also now use 3D reconstructions to help plan complex surgeries. Robotic surgery, which relies on accurate imaging, is becoming increasingly common. The guesswork that was once part of spinal surgeries is gone.

In the operating room, I can see all the preoperative images on a monitor in addition to seeing what I'm doing at the moment. In fact, for some surgeries, I use a very sophisticated version of a computer game console, including the joystick. It's sort of like playing a video game, except instead of racking up points, I rack up extremely accurate procedures.

What all these developments mean for patients is that surgery can often be avoided. When it is necessary, I know exactly where to go on the spine. The procedures are safer, less painful, have a much faster recovery time, and are a lot more likely to help.

AVOIDING THE COST OF CHRONIC BACK PAIN

According to the World Health Organization, 80 percent or more of all adults will experience back pain at some point. Most will have an acute episode and get over it within a few weeks, but for about 20 percent, back pain becomes chronic. Back pain that doesn't go away is a huge burden for both individuals and the medical system. It's one of the top reasons people miss work or can't do all the normal activities of daily living, and it's the second-leading cause of disability. Back pain is also hugely expensive. Americans spend nearly $50 billion a year on direct treatment costs for back pain. Another $100 billion in indirect costs comes from lost productivity and wages and other expenses.

Back pain isn't just costly in economic terms. It has a major impact on your life that can't be measured in dollars and cents. Back pain costs you a lot of personal time. It's the third-leading cause of visits to the doctor. It's a major cause of time off work—and enough time off work can force you into a different job or derail your career track. You might end up on disability or forced into early retirement. You could put a number on those costs, but you can't put a number on missed vacations or time you spend in pain instead of with your friends and family. You can't put a number on the way back pain can take you away from the things you enjoy and even limit you in the activities of daily living.

In this book, I'll teach you how changes to your diet and lifestyle can help keep your back pain from becoming chronic and requiring surgery. I'll explain the nonsurgical alternatives, such as physical therapy, stem cell injections, and even acupuncture. If you do need surgery, I'll explain why, what the options are, and help you prepare for a good outcome and quick recovery. I'll also discuss specific types of minimally invasive surgery in detail, so you know what approach is best for you and what to expect. And I'll discuss the pros and cons of the latest precision laser surgical and robotic techniques.

My goal with this book is to educate you to be an effective advocate for your own wellness. I want to give you the power to affect your diagnosis of chronic back pain in a positive way. When other approaches haven't worked, the minimally invasive surgical option is often the best choice, even if you've had previous back surgery or have been told you're not a good candidate for surgery. Today, we can offer tremendous hope for helping chronic back pain and returning you to a full and active life.

CHAPTER 1

Getting to Pain-Free

My patient John had a long and circuitous path to curing his back pain—it took him around the world until it ended in my office in Virginia. John was a very successful businessman in his seventies. He was still active in his company and traveled a lot for business. He also made plenty of time to enjoy his hobbies of competitive ice dancing and mountain climbing. Unfortunately, pinched nerves in the lumbar (lower back) section of his spine, caused by arthritis and scoliosis, were severely hampering his activities.

John came to see me because he was searching for a solution to his constant pain. I told him we could do surgery on his entire spine, but it would have a long recovery period and leave him with very little flexibility. His ice dancing days would be over. I also told him that a smaller, much less invasive surgery that could help quite a bit was also possible. He listened carefully and then went searching the world for more opinions. He went to Baltimore to consult with some famous sports doctors. He went to Switzerland and got opinions there. He went to doctors in Germany. He came back to me, and I repeated what I told him before. After that, he went to another doctor and had a surgery that didn't help.

Finally, he came back to me and we went ahead with the minimally invasive surgery (MIS) I had originally proposed. He was better in two weeks. He was back to ice dancing at six weeks. Three months after that, he sent me a picture of himself on top of a mountain. He and his wife noted that he stood taller and that he felt and looked younger. He still feels this way years later.

John is a bit out of the ordinary in his ability to travel the world, seeking opinions on his back pain, but in other respects, he's very typical of my patients. They've been in constant pain from spinal issues for a long time, they've tried other solutions, sometimes including surgery, and then they come to me. I do a minimally invasive procedure, relieve their pain, and have them back on their feet and back to their life within a few weeks.

To understand why, we need to back up a little.

THE UPPER END OF THE CURVE

The average medical student gets about an hour of nutrition training during their schooling. That's what I got, too, but something I learned in that hour stayed with me. I was told that the recommended daily allowance (RDA) for nutrients is designed by a committee so that the majority of healthy people who get that amount will avoid disease. That completely spun me around. Before that, I thought that if you got the RDA, you'd be healthy. But the RDA doesn't optimize health—it just helps you avoid disease. That's something completely different. I'm not into avoiding disease. I'm into optimizing health.

WHAT THE RDA MEANS

The Food and Nutrition Board of the Institute of Medicine, National Academy of Sciences (a nongovernment, nonprofit organization), sets the national guidelines for adequate dietary intake of nutrients. The board sets the research-based Recommended Dietary Allowance (RDA) for nutrients. The RDA is defined as the average daily level of intake sufficient to meet the nutrient requirements of nearly all (at least 97 percent) healthy people. In other words, it sets the minimum amount to avoid deficiencies, not the amount for optimal health or the amounts for people who aren't healthy.

I wanted to learn to be at the upper end of the bell curve, where people are healthiest. I didn't want to be just in the middle and certainly not at the lower end.

The science of optimal health drew me in. I still vividly remember browsing through the library stacks when I was in medical school and running across a book by someone who described the benefits of interval training and high-intensity exercise—thirty years before CrossFit and other fitness programs became the rage. The same thing happened with fish oil. Researchers thirty years ago were describing the benefits of omega-3 fatty acids, but fish oil supplements didn't really exist. The researchers could only recommend eating sardines and anchovy sandwiches.

As a surgeon, I continued to follow the research in the realms of nutrition and human performance. I became convinced that nutrition is key to avoiding and healing spine problems. In my practice today as a spine surgeon, I find that most people can get better nonoperatively if they do the right exercises, lose weight, and change their diet. Sometimes, at the end of the day, I realize that I didn't recommend a single patient for surgery. They were all getting better with nonoperative approaches.

For those who need more help, we offer medication, injections, stem cells, and platelet-rich plasma (PRP) treatments. I usually see surgery as a last resort, used only when other treatments haven't helped. When it is needed, I almost always do it with minimally invasive techniques and advanced technology. I was one of the first surgeons on the east coast to use artificial discs for lower back surgery. I was also one of the first to use stem cells and robotic surgery.

The surgery I did on John was a direct lateral interbody fusion. One of his discs had collapsed. Using just a three-inch incision on his side, I was able to remove the damaged disc and replace it with an artificial one. The procedure is similar to putting in a shim. This opened a space for the nerve, took away the leg pain, and realigned part of the spine to give him better balance. The key was figuring out exactly where the artificial disc should go.

John was in the hospital for just a few days. In the old days, he would have been in bed for three months or would have had a plaster cast from his knees to his armpits and would have had a much bigger surgery. Today, we hold the fused discs in place with tiny screws that stabilize it. My patients are generally up and walking by the next day, and often the same day. As soon as the incision heals, they start physical therapy. In John's case, that was water rehab, so he could exercise with less pressure on the spine. From there, he graduated to regular physical therapy that focused on building his muscles and getting his core back in shape.

INSURANCE COVERAGE

Health insurance doesn't always cover some of the procedures I do. Even though they're safe and very effective, they're on the cutting edge (so to speak), and there haven't been enough formal studies to make the insurance companies always have to pay for them. That's a problem because the cost can be high. But the cost of not doing the surgery can be high, too. I have a patient who started her own business after retiring from the military. After seven or eight years of struggling, the company is now doing very well. She has 350 employees and revenues of over $30 million. She was in a lot of pain and needed the sort of surgery that would get her back to running the company quickly, but her insurer wasn't willing to pay for it. She told me to put her on the operating room schedule, because as a CEO, she knew that sometimes you have to put your health first and just pay the bill. In the end, after surgery, she was able to negotiate with her insurer for reimbursement. She was back at work a week after the surgery; three months later she was completely pain-free.

GETTING YOUR LIFE BACK

I keep a picture of Ginny in her wedding dress in my office. When she first came to me, she was twenty-six and had been in miserable back pain for several years. She could barely get up from the couch, much less get to class or to work. Her social life was nonexistent. The doctors she saw couldn't figure out why her back hurt so much. They also told her that even if they could, she was too young for spine surgery.

She came to me for help. We tried nonoperative approaches

for a year, but they didn't help much. I ended up testing her discs and found that three of them had big tears, even though MRIs didn't show any herniations. We talked about what to do. She said, "Everybody else says I'm too young for surgery. They want me to wait twenty years, and then they'll think about doing it. I'm already twenty-six. They want me to give up another half of my life while I wait for something that might help." We decided to go ahead with fusion surgery. It went very well—Ginny was pain-free and active again for the first time in years.

The next time I saw Ginny was about eighteen months later. She was off her pain meds, active, married, and six months pregnant. She told me, "Before I had surgery, I basically went to doctor's visits, therapy, and home. I couldn't do anything more. After surgery, within a few months, I was up and around and able to spend time with my friends. I got back to school and ended up meeting my husband." Why was she in my office? She wanted to know if the surgery affected her ability to have a normal delivery. I told her it didn't, and she wouldn't need an elective C-section. Back surgery turned Ginny from a depressed hermit back into a vibrant young woman with an active life ahead of her.

And then there's the problem of depression. Constant pain is just depressing. Constant pain where all you can do is lie on the couch and watch daytime TV is even more depressing. Powerful pain medicine is helpful in the very short run, but it quickly stops being very effective. That means escalating the dose and running the risk of getting you dependent on the drug—or even addicted to it.

Our attitude about operating on younger people has changed. If you're in pain at a time in your life when you should be active, and if other approaches have been tried and didn't work, surgery makes sense. In the past, when back surgery was a very big operation and had a long recovery period and when nonoperative approaches weren't as sophisticated, waiting had some logic. But today, I prefer to wait just a year or two to give nonoperative approaches a good chance to help. If they don't, why should someone be condemned to twenty years of pain and life limitations when minimally invasive surgery can help?

NONOPERATIVE OPTIONS

Over-the-counter nonsteroidal anti-inflammatory drugs (NSAIDs) such as naproxen (Naprosyn) and ibuprofen (Advil) can be helpful for minor back pain, but they're not much use beyond that. Prescription NSAIDs such as celecoxib (Celebrex) are more effective, but carry other risks; some can even increase the risk of a heart attack. We've come to see how dangerous narcotic drugs such as oxycodone can be. Whenever possible, I prefer to treat back pain with a minimal amount of drugs and a maximum amount of other nonoperative therapies.

Physical therapy is the main nonoperative treatment for back pain. It gets you back in motion and helps prevent another episode of back pain. In physical therapy, you're taught how to improve your posture and how to avoid another injury by learning to move correctly. A physical therapist also teaches you how to do exercises to strengthen your core—the quadriceps and the hamstrings (thighs), gluteal muscles (butt), abdomen, and back. A strong core that helps keep your back stable is key to preventing another injury. Doing the exercises regularly at home, not just in a therapy session, is crucial for success. Physical therapy teaches you active exercises that are essential to rebuild your muscles.

Too many of us don't exercise much during the week. We sit way too much, and we forget that we don't have the resilience of a fifteen-year-old. We have to actively stay in shape. Physical therapy can also help you get rid of bad posture and body imbalances. If you've been limping for a while because of sciatica (severe leg pain coming from the lower back), for instance, you might have subconsciously forgotten how to walk correctly. That can lead to throwing the rest of your body out of balance. You might be walking crooked, with your neck and jaw jutting forward. Now you've also got neck pain or even a disc herniation in your neck. Physical therapy can help you get back into balance and walking correctly.

A nonoperative modality that works well for some patients

is chiropractic treatment. In the short-term, hands-on treatments from a skilled chiropractor, such as simple massage, stretching, and spinal manipulation can relieve pain and get you back to normal activity sooner than not doing it. A lot of doctors will say that chiropractic treatment doesn't help, but the evidence in its favor, including some recent excellent studies, is convincing. I don't hesitate to recommend it when I think it will help.

Acupuncture and dry needling have also been shown to help back pain. Traditional Chinese acupuncture uses very thin, sterile needles inserted along energy meridians to relieve the pain. In dry needling, the needles are also very thin. They're inserted into trigger points—tender areas in muscles that are like painful knots—to relax the area and relieve pain. The tiny needles don't contain any medication (that's why they're "dry"). In skilled hands, this is a very effective technique for quick pain relief.

Other passive forms of therapy include ultrasound, TENS units, and infrared light. Ultrasound uses low-frequency sound waves sent through the skin above the painful area. The sound waves make the soft tissue vibrate, which creates heat and increases blood flow. The improved blood flow relaxes tight muscles and reduces pain. Sometimes we also use a topical cream that helps reduce inflammation. The ultrasound helps drive the cream further into the skin and makes it more effective.

TENS stands for transcutaneous electrical nerve stimulation. TENS units work by sending very mild electrical impulses (tiny shocks) through the skin. The impulses help block pain signals from reaching the brain. You can get TENS treatment from a physical therapist using a professional-grade unit to deliver the impulses. Some of my patients find that small, portable units designed for home use help them.

Infrared light and some forms of low-level laser therapy in specific wavelengths can be helpful. Infrared light and low-level lasers provide light without heat, which can help stimulate cell repair and collagen growth, improve mitochondrial function within cells, decrease inflammation, and enhance healing. Some medical clinics and PTs offer this form of treatment.

STEROIDS AND EPIDURAL INJECTIONS

Let's say you have a serious flare-up of back pain from a muscle spasm or pinched nerve in your lower back. Ibuprofen and other NSAIDs aren't going to help. Instead, I'll prescribe oral steroids, drugs that are very good for bringing down inflammation. The problem is that when you take a pill, it goes throughout the entire body. It decreases the local inflammation, but it also affects the rest of the body, including your liver and kidneys. In the long-term, oral steroids can cause bad side effects; not everybody can take them. Using them short-term for back pain is usually safe.

If oral steroids don't work well for you, we need to consider an epidural injection instead. This means injecting the steroid directly into the space outside the dura, the sac around the nerve roots that contains cerebrospinal fluid (the fluid that bathes the nerve roots). That sounds painful, but before we give you the main injection, we numb the area with a small needle and a dose of local anesthetic. The procedure is very safe.

When we inject the steroid exactly where it's needed, it works well and the effect is limited to that area. The steroid helps calm down the inflammation directly where it is, which relieves the pressure on the spinal nerves and helps alleviate the pain. Often the injection is all the patient needs. It calms the nerves down enough to let them heal and the pain goes away.

When we use an injection instead of steroid pills, it's like the difference between putting ice on your ankle for a sprain and drinking iced tea for it. The injection works immediately, as opposed to steroid pills, which take a day or more to start kicking in.

Injections aren't just therapeutic—they also help us diagnose back pain. Sometimes a patient is in so much pain that I can't be sure from the X-rays and other tests if they have a disc problem or something else. A good way to tell is to do a local injection of a numbing medication such as

Novocaine or lidocaine into the suspect area. It's like going to the dentist, where you get a shot to numb just the tooth that needs it. I inject the area where I think the problem is and see what happens. If the medicine works and relieves the pain temporarily, we're closer to knowing what's causing it and what to do about it.

There are many types of injections, such as facet injections, nerve root blocks, intra-articular injections, to name a few. Each of them is used for a specific problem or in an attempt to discover an underlying cause of pain—to help in both the diagnosis and treatment of pain.

> More recently, instead of using steroids as the medicine being injected, PRP (platelet rich plasma), PPP (platelet poor plasma), or stem cells are being used for some of these injections. Initial results are looking promising. Many patients are feeling improved symptoms, and larger clinical studies are underway as well.

Patients always ask me, "How long's this injection going to work, doc?" I say, "Well, the medicine will probably be out of your system in a day or two. That's long enough to help the inflammation and get you walking around again. Once the inflammation is taken care of, your body can start the healing process." The injection can jumpstart the recovery process. When the inflammation is improved, there is often less pain. Even if the medicine is gone in a couple of days, the injection's effects may be long-lasting. I often give a patient an injection or a short series of injections and never see them again, or see them only down the road if the pain comes back. (I'll talk more about how helpful injections can be in chapter 4.)

WEIGHT LOSS AND NUTRITION

I'm a surgeon, but in my practice, I help patients do everything they can to avoid back surgery by optimizing their wellness. For a majority of my patients, that means losing weight and improving their nutrition. I'll go into weight loss and nutrition for healing back problems in detail in chapter 4. For now, I'll just say that if you're overweight, you're putting a lot of extra stress on your spine and your joints, especially your knees and hips. Losing weight is probably the single most effective thing you can do to stop your back pain.

Overweight or not, improving your nutritional status is also key to stopping back pain. For instance, many patients recommended for back surgery turn out to have low levels of vitamin C and vitamin D. In my clinic over the last few years, I've tested over 300 people sequentially for their vitamin D levels. Eighty percent were suboptimal (under 50 on a normal range of 30 to 100), and half of them weren't even in the normal range. A quarter of them were just barely normal.

We're all just not getting enough vitamin D because we're

not getting enough sunlight and we're not eating correctly. Vitamin D is crucial for building and maintaining strong bones. Having low vitamin D levels may be one reason we're having more osteopenia and osteoporosis and the back trouble that comes with them. I take an optimized dose of 15,000 units of vitamin D every day, based on my lab test values. I recommend vitamin D to my patients. When they start taking extra vitamin D, in the amount their lab work suggests, their achy bones and joint pain often get a lot better. Surprisingly, if they're depressed, the depression often gets better, too. Some of my patients are able to stop taking antidepressants.

Higher doses of vitamin D are a bit controversial, but they're generally safe and almost certainly can't hurt you. A 2015 study in the *Journal of the American Medical Association* says that almost everyone should be getting at least 5,000 units a day, which is far more than you can get by sun exposure and diet. My feeling is that testing for vitamin D levels is inexpensive and easy—it's just a simple blood test. The vitamin pills are inexpensive as well. If you have back pain, taking the optimal dose of vitamin D is cheap and easy. It's certainly worth trying to see if it helps. How much vitamin D you specifically should take will be personalized based upon your laboratory tests and clinical situation.

Fish oil, which contains omega-3 fatty acids, can be extremely helpful for reducing inflammation without the side effects of NSAIDs and steroids. The key to getting the benefits of omega-3s is having a good ratio of them to other dietary fats. The standard American diet is unfortunately very high in omega-6 fatty acids, which are found in the cheap, nutritionally empty vegetable oils used in processed foods. When the dietary balance is skewed in favor of omega-6 fatty acids, inflammation is increased.

When you stop to think about it, in our diet, we get most of our omega-3 fatty acids from grass. The grass of the ocean are plankton. The plankton are eaten by fatty fish such as salmon, who store the omega-3s found in plankton in their fat. On land, grass-fed cattle do basically the same thing, so eating pastured beef is another way to get omega-3s naturally. Green leafy vegetables such as kale contain a lot of omega-3s; so do nuts. To get enough omega-3 fatty acids to reduce inflammation, often you'll need to take supplements, preferably in the form of purified fish oil capsules, until you are able to change your diet (in particular, stopping the use of vegetable oils in your diet).

What you don't want to eat is sugar in any form. There's a simple way to avoid sugar: Don't eat anything white. (I'll explain why in detail in chapter 3.)

TRACTION NO MORE

Years ago, if your back went out from a disc problem, your

doctor would put you in traction. While in traction, you'd lie in bed for days or weeks on end, attached to a hanging weight at the foot of the bed. The idea was to physically stretch out the spine and relieve the pressure on the affected disc. Light traction for short periods can be helpful for a pinched nerve in the neck, but we now know that it's not only useless for back pain, it can actually be harmful by immobilizing you and weakening your muscles.

EXERCISE

Exercise is huge for helping back pain. Both aerobic fitness (heart health) and anaerobic fitness (muscle strength) are absolutely central to preventing back pain to begin with, treating it, and keeping it from coming back. When you're strong and fit, you stand up straight and have strong core muscles that stabilize your back. Unfortunately, most people today spend a lot of time sitting, which leads to poor posture and muscle imbalances, such as contractures and hamstring tightness. In terms of your health, chronic sitting is the new smoking. You need lots of exercise to counteract the effects. A lot of so-called ergonomic chairs don't help. You might be comfortable when you sit, but sitting on any sort of chair is the underlying problem. I suggest sitting, at least some of the time, on an exercise ball to keep your core muscles engaged, or pretend you are sitting on a balance ball. You have to have good posture on the exercise ball, because otherwise you'll fall off. Back in college, my piano instructor, Father Jerome, taught me how to sit on the piano bench by sitting on the front third of it, with my feet directly in front of me. My core was gently balanced, I could reach the whole keyboard without straining, and my upper body wasn't tired after playing for an hour or two.

My other recommendation is to get out of the chair as much as possible. If you can, stand up and walk around when you're on the phone. Set your watch alarm to go off every half hour to remind you to stand up at your desk and move around a bit, just enough to get the blood moving but not enough to wreck your concentration or interrupt your work.

I teach my patients how to do a simple squat using their desk chair. All you have to do is stand up from your chair, then bring your butt down again slowly, as if you're going to sit down. Just touch your butt to the chair and stand up again slowly. Do that five to ten times and then get back to work. The squat movement engages your lower back, thigh, and gluteal (butt) muscles, which is good for strengthening them. It also reminds your muscles to stay balanced and not sit hunched over. When you sit with a good balance in your lower back, it automatically throws your shoulders back where they belong and it keeps your head well balanced over your neck and shoulders. Squats also get the blood flowing better back out of your legs and into the rest of your body. We know from studies that doing five squats every half hour is much better than doing 40 squats once a day.

You can do simple exercises like squats every day without taking a lot of time, working up a sweat, or needing any special equipment. If you're sent for physical therapy for your back pain, your therapist will teach you how to do these exercises correctly.

Now that you have a good idea of what we can do to help your back pain, let's get down to the real question: What's causing your back pain? That's going to take all of the next chapter to explain.

CHAPTER 2

What's Causing Your Back Pain?

Back pain has a lot of possible causes, but the causes that bring you to a surgeon's office are almost always related to nerve pain from damage to the spine. If you're having nerve pain, chances are good we can help you without operating, but sometimes surgery is the best option.

ROWING AGAINST THE TIDE

One of my patients was a twenty-two-year-old competitive rower on her Ivy League college team. For 18 months, she had been in so much pain from a back injury that she couldn't row. She also couldn't sit—she had to stand in the back of the classroom and couldn't get much schoolwork done. Her grades were suffering to the point where she was warned about not graduating on time. Nonoperative treatments weren't helping. I was able to pinpoint the source of her pain and do a minimally invasive fusion and stabilization procedure. The surgery was very successful—she was off her pain meds almost immediately and was able to get back to class and her sports.

SCIATICA

Sciatica is an old-fashioned term for the pain that comes from a pinched nerve in the lower back. Lumbago is an even more old-fashioned term for this pain. The medical term for sciatica is radiculopathy, meaning pain caused by irritation or compression of the nerve as it comes out of the spinal column. Radiculopathy can happen in any part of the spine, but it's most common in the lower back and neck. Another name for sciatica is a pinched nerve; it's also sometimes called a slipped disc. Radiculopathy is the most common form of nerve-related back pain.

In sciatica, the pain starts in your butt muscles and shoots down the sciatic nerve at the back of your leg. If you bend or sit too much or straighten out the leg, it hurts more because these positions stretch and irritate the nerve. Even coughing or sneezing makes it hurt more. You have trouble walking because whenever you're moving, the pain shoots down your leg. In addition to or sometimes instead of pain, you might have weakness, tingling, or numbness in your leg. (If the pinched nerve is in your neck, you'll have pain, weakness, tingling, and numbness in your arm.)

What's causing all this misery? It's probably because the rubbery, disc-shaped tissue that acts as a shock absorber between each vertebra in your spine is damaged. Spinal discs are sort of like jelly donuts. They have a tough, outer core and a softer, gelatinous inner core. When a disc gets compressed or injured or just partially worn out from wear and tear, you can have a disc herniation, where the soft inner core is so squished that it bulges out through the tough, outer core. It's like the way a bald tire bulges and eventually blows out. The problem is that there's no room in the spinal area for the bulge. Like a rock in your shoe, it irritates the area and causes pain. If the bulge is pressing on the nerve that comes out of that vertebra in the lower back, you have leg pain, numbness, weakness, and tingling.

Sometimes the pain is a result of degenerative disc disease, which causes the disc to weaken and move too much, which then can irritate the nerve roots in the area. Sometimes degenerative disc disease can cause bone spurs that press on the nerve. And sometimes a worn-out disc just causes back pain, just as arthritis of the knee makes the knee hurt without pressing on a nerve.

A lot of pain is related to the inflammation of the nerve that comes from the affected area. It's being punched, so it gets angry and hurts. If we can calm that nerve down, even if we don't do anything about the bulging disc or bone spur that's causing the problem to begin with, the nerve stops being angry. The symptoms get better gradually and may not ever come back.

However, if you don't get better nonoperatively, a minimally invasive surgery to take the pressure off the nerve often helps. The surgery is like taking a small stone out of your shoe when it's making your foot hurt. Once the stone is removed, the foot is no longer irritated.

The good news is that approximately eight out of ten people feel better nonoperatively in the first eight weeks after an attack of sciatica. To be a little more precise, six out of ten will feel better in the first six weeks and eight out of ten will feel better in eight weeks. If you're not much better in eight weeks or more, or if the pain is truly horrible, that's when we start thinking about doing surgery.

Standard nonoperative treatment helps the vast majority of people with sciatica. As long as you're not having progressive weakness and if the pain isn't so bad that you're just incapacitated by it, then usually I'll want you to wait it out by taking nonprescription anti-inflammatory drugs such as ibuprofen or naprosyn. If you need it, we can use a prescription NSAID such as indomethacin or try steroids for a short time. Just as important is resting for a few days. You want to decrease movement so the nerve isn't being irritated all the time, but that doesn't mean taking to your bed for a week. Just take it easy for a few days and try to lie down when you can. When you have a disc that's causing sciatic pain, you'll need to change up your activities and take it easy for a bit. After the first few days, you should get back to your usual daily activities as much as you can, but you're not going to be running and jumping for a while or doing any other activity that keeps irritating the nerve.

Between the drugs and the rest, the worst of the inflammation is usually over in a few days. If it's not, we can try an injection of steroids or a local anesthetic directly into the affected area.

Once the worst is over, I'll have you start some gentle exercise and stretching for a week or two and then send you for physical therapy. As your pain gets better, physical therapy can help you relearn how to move to protect your spine and balance out your muscle strength.

If surgery is necessary, the usual treatment would be a microdiscectomy. The goal of the surgery is to shrink down the bulging disc or remove the herniated portion of it that's pinching the nerve. Another treatment would be a laminotomy, which is very similar to a discectomy—in fact, the two terms are often used interchangeably. In this procedure, we remove part of the lamina (the outer "roof" of the vertebra that covers the nerves) and make a little window in it. That lets me get down to where the nerve is and decompress it by moving it away from the bulging disc. At the same time, I can remove the herniated section of the disc.

With minimally invasive surgery (MIS) techniques, microdiscectomy and laminotomy can be done on an outpatient basis. The outcomes for both are usually excellent. Once the incision and spine have healed up over the next few weeks, you can get back to your full activity level.

SPINAL STENOSIS

Another cause of sciatica is spinal stenosis, a narrowing of the spinal canal in the lower back region that makes the disc bulge and put pressure on the nerve roots. Spinal stenosis usually goes along with spinal arthritis. To a degree, it's a normal part of aging; it's commonly seen in people over age sixty. It causes more pinching than a herniated disc because the whole spinal canal in the area is narrowed. Spinal stenosis happens mostly in the lower back and the lumbar spine.

The common symptoms of all the nerves being pinched, as opposed to one or two nerves in sciatica, are an achiness that starts in the lower back and goes down one or both legs. It happens when you stand because then the curve in your back pinches in on the nerves. Your legs feel very achy and heavy; you probably can't walk more than a block or two. To un-pinch the nerves, you can sit down or bend forward to take the pressure off your back.

The treatment for spinal stenosis is pretty much the same as for sciatica—anti-inflammatories, rest, and physical therapy. Epidural injections often help quite a bit. If nonoperative approaches don't help, then we can do surgery to take the pressure off the nerves.

SPONDYLOLISTHESIS

Another cause of leg pain from a back problem is spondylolisthesis (pronounced SPON-dill-oh-lis-THEE-sis). Literally, it means "spine stepping," where one vertebra slips forward on the other, so your spine looks like a staircase instead of a column. The vertebrae of the spine are stacked on top of each other. There's a tunnel—the spinal canal—that the nerves go through. If one vertebra starts slipping forward, it narrows the tunnel and makes the space for the nerves a lot smaller. That compresses them and causes irritation, inflammation, and pain. If the bone slips, the facet joints in the back of the spine, which link one vertebra to another, get enlarged from arthritis and press on the nerves. The slipping bone can also cause stenosis and pain.

Isthmic spondylolisthesis can happen when you have microfractures in the narrow part of the lamina called the pars interarticularis. The fractures can be from wear and tear or from osteoporosis. The fracture lets one vertebra collapse onto the one below it and pinch the nerves. At first, it may not pinch much, so you may not even know it is happening. But as it progresses, you may start to have symptoms. You might not have any pain initially, just some hamstring tightness. Later on, you can get back pain or leg pain similar to a disc herniation.

Damage to the pars interarticularis is fairly common among teenage football players and gymnasts, but they often don't have any symptoms when it first occurs. It's only when they hit their forties, fifties, or even older that the old injury catches up to them, and they start having problems.

The treatment is to stabilize the sliding vertebrae and take the pressure off the nerves. We almost always have to do a fusion to stabilize and realign the spine. The surgery usually involves a surgical cage to hold the bone in place while it fuses. Sometimes we also remove the disc and replace it with an artificial one. I use minimally invasive techniques for the surgery, so the procedure usually takes about ninety minutes and involves only a night or two in the hospital. The recovery time is fairly short. (I'll describe it in depth in chapter 7.) The surgery is usually very successful no matter what age you are or how long you've had the problem. I did a fusion on a teenage boy about fifteen years ago and he went on to become a professional triathlete. We sponsor an annual event for spine care awareness that features a 5K run. He's usually leading the pack.

NECK AND ARM PAIN

When a disc in the cervical (neck) area gets damaged

or herniated, you get pain or numbness down your neck and into your shoulder blade or arm. It's like sciatica, but in your upper body. Sometimes the symptoms are mild, causing just numbness in the thumb and first and second fingers. Sometimes the symptoms are mistaken for the hand pain and numbness of carpal tunnel syndrome.

Cervical pinched nerves are mostly a result of wear and tear on the vertebrae. Posture plays a role, though. If you slouch in a chair a lot, your face is thrust forward and your chin is raised. That puts a lot of pressure on the neck and stretches out the muscles in the front of the neck. When the pressure is imbalanced like that, the nerves can get pinched.

As with leg pain from sciatica, the initial treatment is to calm down the inflammation. This is the one condition where old-fashioned traction can be helpful. We'll use gentle traction to pull up on the head to open up the foramina, which are the openings where the nerves come out of the spinal column. Otherwise, treatment is very similar to sciatica. We can calm the cervical nerves down nonoperatively in 60 to 80 percent of patients.

If the pinched nerve doesn't get better, we can do surgery to take the pressure off of it. Often, then means removing the damaged disc and replacing it with an artificial one.

SCOLIOSIS: CURVATURE OF THE SPINE

Scoliosis is an abnormal sideways curve in the spine, a problem that usually develops in preteens and teenagers. If the curve is mild, it may not need any treatment. But if the curve is big, it can cause real problems by reducing the space for your heart and lungs. You can't breathe as well and your heart doesn't work as well, to the point of limiting your activity and even shortening your life. Even if the curve is mild, it can cause the nerves on one side of the spine to be compressed and lead to pain, deformity, and disability.

When it looks like the curve is going to get worse as the child grows, surgery may be the solution. It can stabilize and realign the spine before the curvature starts causing problems. It also helps the child stand up straight and be normally active. We usually do the surgery during adolescence, around age fifteen or sixteen or sometimes older. Sometimes scoliosis happens with spinal degeneration over time. That might be much later on in life, in your fifties or sixties.

Sometimes the procedure can't be done as minimally invasive surgery because it has to include the entire portion of the spine that's abnormally curved. It's definitely become much more precise, however. We no longer need to operate on the entire spine or put you in a body cast for weeks on end. Today, we can use hooks and screws to hold each spot in place and fuse it into its new position. The surgery is easier on the patient, and the recovery time is a lot shorter.

There are some newer, minimally invasive and robotic procedures and techniques that can be used to treat some types of scoliosis. The field is continuing to advance. It is possible that you may be a good candidate for these techniques if you need surgery.

FLAT BACK SYNDROME

When you look at the spine from the side, you see it's got an S shape, with curves at the neck and the lower back. The two curves balance each other out to let you stand up straight, with your head centered over your hips. In flat back syndrome, the curve in the lower back gets smaller and flatter, usually because of worn-out discs and arthritis in the spine. When the normal lumbar curvature is lost, that puts you off balance. You lean your head forward and start having trouble standing upright and walking normally. That's very fatiguing and causes a lot of back pain.

We can operate to help a flat back. It can be a very big surgery, but more often, we do a smaller surgery to reconstruct just the bottom part of the spine and restore a good part of the curve. If that's where the nerves are being pinched, we take the pressure off, realign the vertebrae, and fuse them at a better angle.

For many patients, however, there's a simpler solution. We give them a walking stick. This may not be ideal for a younger patient, but for patients in their seventies or older who don't want a big surgery and aren't that active anymore, a Moses staff can help take the pressure off the lower back and let them walk a lot better.

TRAUMA

Trauma can be as severe as a paralyzing injury to the spinal cord itself or as mild as a bad bruise to the spine from falling off a skateboard. In my practice, I see the full range. The most common traumatic injury I see, however, it a fractured vertebra in the thoracolumbar region. That's where the thoracic (chest) vertebrae, which are very rigid, and the lumbar (lower back) vertebrae, which are more flexible, come together. The usual cause is a car accident where the vehicle comes to a sudden stop. You rapidly bend forward and then back, which compresses the spine in that area, to the point where the bone fractures. Small compression fractures usually heal by themselves if we put you in a brace or a cast, but some of these injuries are more serious fractures that are unstable. If we don't treat you surgically, you could end up disabled with a lot of pain and loss of function.

We want the surgery to take pressure off the nerve and stabilize the spine in the area. We don't want to immobilize you afterward by putting you in a cast, because that means a big loss of muscle tone in the area, just when you want your back to be strong. With minimally invasive surgery, we can use cages and screws to decompress the area and hold it in alignment. The surgery takes less time and has less risk of complications than doing an open procedure. You have less pain afterward, a shorter hospital stay, and the time you have to spend immobilized afterward is much shorter. You can start physical therapy and get back to your normal life much sooner.

WILL THE PAIN COME BACK?

Most back pain needs only nonoperative treatments and some patience. After eight to ten weeks, most patients are feeling fine and are back to their normal activities. After such a painful experience, however, they are naturally worried that back pain will strike them again.

It might. If you have a significant episode of back pain, the odds within a year of having another episode that puts you down for a week are high. How high? In my view, nobody really knows. The scientific studies report ranges anywhere from 30 to 75 percent. Whatever the real rate of recurrence is, odds that high are a good reason for following through with your physical therapy. When you've learned how to strengthen your core muscles and how to move to avoid injury, your odds of having another episode are lower.

Many of my patients have episodes of back pain once or twice a year that last for just a few days or even less. If you get over the pain quickly and the rest of the time you're able to do what you want and need to do, that's acceptable. You probably won't ever need surgery. Only a small minority of my patients don't get better with nonoperative treatments.

Having nonoperative treatments for back pain will usually make those episodes shorter and more tolerable. Each time you're treated, you'll also be reminded of what you need to do to avoid back pain in the future. You have a chance to make sure you don't have any bad posture habits, to be reminded to do your back exercises and exercise in general, and to use the right body mechanics when lifting something heavy. Most importantly, you'll be reminded that losing weight and eating a healthy diet are key to avoiding back pain. So key, in fact, that I'll spend the next chapter explaining why.

CHAPTER 3

Your Wellness Landscape

I'm a surgeon, but I don't like to operate on patients unless I'm certain that surgery is the best and only solution to their back pain. Often, it isn't. The solution to getting their back well is getting the rest of their body well.

My first realization of this fundamental idea came from one of my earliest patients, a retired Air Force officer. The colonel loved golf. All he wanted to do in his retirement was play golf and make golf clubs. The problem was, his back and his hands had become so stiff that he couldn't do either anymore. He couldn't even hold a club.

He came to me for help, thinking it was a spine problem. I examined him and didn't find anything specifically wrong with his spine. I didn't see anything that surgery could help. Then I remembered back to a lecture from my medical school days on the role of fatty acids in health. When the fatty acids are imbalanced, inflammation—stiffness, swelling, joint pain—can occur. Perhaps that was causing the pain and stiffness the colonel was experiencing. He told me he ate a lot of fried foods, which meant he was eating a lot of a type of fatty acid called omega-6. What he wasn't eating was the beneficial type of fatty acid found in fish, nuts, avocados, and pastured beef and eggs, called omega-3. (I'll go into the details of the fatty acids a little later in this chapter.) Ideally, a good diet has lots of omega-3s and not too much in the way of omega-6s. The colonel's was the opposite.

I asked him to start taking 5,000 units a day of fish oil and asked him to cut back on the fried foods. About four months later, he returned and told me his joints had stopped aching and he was feeling a lot better. He was back to making golf clubs and back to playing golf. He was able to hit balls out of the rough again, without the club flying out of his hands. Simply by changing his diet and reaching a much better balance of fatty acids, he was able to stop being my patient and return to the thing he loved.

The dramatic improvement in the colonel's health made me think that I needed to know more about nutrition beyond the basics I had been taught in medical school.

WHY FATS ARE GOOD

For years, we doctors bought the low-fat propaganda. We believed that fat was bad for you and that it was the root of all health evils. Boy, were we wrong.

Let's start with the basic nutritional fact that your body needs fat from your diet. In fact, you need fat so much that some types of fat are called essential fatty acids. Essential means you have to have them, just as you have to have vitamins from your diet or from supplements. You need fat from your diet for every body function, including providing energy, making and repairing the membranes that enclose your cells, and building the hormones that direct your metabolism.

Doctors are always telling their patients to stay away from "bad" saturated fats and to eat more "good" unsaturated fats. Saturated fats are mostly found in animal foods; they're solid at room temperature. Unsaturated fats are mostly found in plant foods; they're liquid (oils) at room temperature. For example, butter, lard, chicken fat, beef fat, and other animal fats are saturated, while olive oil, walnut oil, coconut oil, fish oil, and others are unsaturated fats.

Why does this matter? It doesn't.

What matters is the ratio of essential fatty acids in your diet. Why? Because you have about 20 different fatty acids in your body, but they're all made from just two essential fatty acids: linoleic acid, better known as omega-6 fatty acid, and linolenic acid, better known as omega-3 fatty acid. Omega-6 (linoleic) and omega-3 (linolenic) fatty acids are essential to your health. You have to get them from your food because your body can't make them. Essential fatty acids are the building blocks for all the other fats in your body. Most foods contain at least some of both essential fatty acids. Some foods are richer sources than others, however.

Omega-3 fatty acids are naturally found in fish and seafood, eggs, whole grains, seeds, nuts, and vegetables. Flaxseeds, flaxseed oil, walnuts, and nut oils are all good sources. Omega-3 fatty acids are plant-based, directly or indirectly. They're found in animal foods, but only when the animal feeds on grass (pastured chicken and beef, for instance) or plankton, the ocean equivalent of grass (wild-caught fish and seafood).

Omega-6 fatty acids are found naturally mostly in seeds and nuts; there's also some in avocados, poultry, and eggs in a good ratio with omega-3 fatty acids. However, in our modern society, omega-6 fatty acids in the diet mostly come from liquid vegetable oils, such as corn oil, canola, sunflower oil, and most of all, soybean oil. Because these cheap, heavily refined oils are used in just about all the baked goods, snack foods, processed foods, and fast food we eat, we end up consuming them in large quantities. Soybean oil may now be making up about 20 percent of all the calories in the standard American diet.

The optimal ratio of omega-6 to omega-3 fatty acids in the diet is 1 to 1; most researchers think that 4 to 1 is as high as it should go. Unfortunately, most Americans today are getting a seriously distorted ratio. Estimates vary, but most of us are probably getting ten to fifteen times or even more omega-6s as omega-3s.

You need omega-6 fatty acids to repair cell damage and as part of the normal inflammation response, but if your omega-6 level is as high as it is for most Americans, your body starts to damage itself through inflammation instead of repair itself.

I'll discuss inflammation in more detail later in this chapter. For now, I'll just say the role of essential fatty acids in inflammation is very complex. The stripped-down version goes like this: your body uses omega-3 and omega-6 fatty acids to make a lot of different hormones and hormone-like signaling chemicals, including prostaglandins and eicosanoids that control inflammation (pain, swelling, redness, stiffness). The pro-inflammatory chemicals mostly use omega-6 fatty acids as building blocks. The anti-inflammatory substances mostly use omega-3 fatty acids as building blocks. If you have a lot of omega-6 fatty acids in your body, they will be preferentially converted to inflammatory substances, quickly and in abundance. At the same time, if you don't have a lot of omega-3 fatty acids, the anti-inflammatory substances have to compete for it with the other body processes that need it. You can't produce anti-inflammatory substances quickly or in large amounts. The inflammatory substances get the upper hand, and you develop chronic inflammation.

By cutting out all the processed food and junk food from your diet, you're sharply reducing the amount of omega-6 fatty acids you eat. If you swap those foods for foods that are high in omega-3 fatty acids, you shift the balance in your body back to a healthier ratio. You reduce inflammation, which means you no longer feel stiff and achy. Your back stops hurting so much.

Diet alone often isn't enough to shift your balance of fatty acids. In addition to making dietary changes, I strongly recommend taking high-quality fish oil supplements every day. For my patients with back pain, I recommend at least 5,000 mg a day.

Additionally, the vegetable oils (actually the seed oils), are highly polyunsaturated, so they have a high risk of oxidation. This becomes a problem with cooking, and with the way the body uses them for energy. The mitochondria create a lot of oxidation products and free radicals with polyunsaturated oils and fats. The saturated fats create many fewer of these problematic free radicals. Current recommendations are returning to using more saturated fats in cooking and in your diet and avoiding the vegetable oils.

WEIGHT LOSS

Being overweight, sometimes even just a little, is the cause of a significant amount of back pain. Particularly if you have a pear shape and carry the extra weight in the abdominal area, it puts a physical strain on the spine. Imagine carrying a bowling ball in a kangaroo pouch on your stomach. You'd be constantly leaning back or hunching forward to take the strain off your back. That puts a lot of strain on your back muscles, vertebrae, and discs. Eventually, they'll start to hurt. In addition, fat around the belly is particularly unhealthy—it's associated with heart disease, diabetes, inflammation, and other serious health issues.

Losing weight is my primary recommendation to most of my patients. I ask them to put some serious effort into weight loss and come back in six months if they're still in pain. The first thing they say at that point is, "How do I do that?"

I used to reply, "Any way you can," but that was before I knew better. Once I educated myself beyond the rudimentary knowledge of nutrition I had from medical school, I was able to give much better advice that has worked for many of my patients. I've learned that the best approach to weight loss is to cut back severely on carbohydrates—sugary and starchy foods. The research tells me that if you want to count anything as a way to lose weight, don't count calories or fat grams. Count carbs.

There's a simpler way to think of it. I say to my patients, "All you need to know can be summed up in one rule: Don't eat anything white."

What am I saying? Get rid of the white flour in your diet, which means don't eat bread, pasta, baked goods. Get rid of the French fries and mashed potatoes. Get rid of the sugar, period. Don't eat processed food or junk food. (It is okay to eat eggs, even if they are white.) And get rid of the oils made from the grains as well.

What can you eat? Eat real food, without nutritional labels or tons of ingredients. Eat lots of vegetables, the leafier and more colorful, the better. High-quality protein and dietary fats—no processed meats. Changing the way you eat can be challenging, of course. But so is having chronic back pain.

THE CARBOHYDRATE-INFLAMMATION CONNECTION

When you eat foods that contain carbohydrates, your

body converts them into glucose, a form of sugar, to use as its primary fuel. The process starts as soon as you put these foods in your mouth. Amylase, an enzyme in your saliva, starts breaking down carbohydrates into glucose the moment you start chewing. As you digest carbohydrates further, they get broken down into more glucose, which is then absorbed into your bloodstream. The more processed the carbohydrates are, the faster they're absorbed, and the quicker the amount of glucose in your circulation—your blood sugar—rises.

To carry glucose into your cells to be used as fuel, your pancreas secretes the hormone insulin. The insulin knocks on the door of the cell (receptors in the cell membrane). The door opens and insulin ushers the glucose in. But if the cell already has all the glucose it needs, or if it has become resistant to the knock, the cell doesn't answer the door. The insulin and the glucose remain in your bloodstream, raising your blood sugar to unhealthy or even diabetic levels. Some of the excess glucose gets stored in your liver, some gets excreted in your urine, but most of it ends up being stored as fat.

The metabolism of sugar and the body's response to it is actually quite complex and involves not only energy but also hormones and fat metabolism. But by doing these relatively simple things, like cutting down on carbohydrates, the body can take care of itself.

UNDERSTANDING INFLAMMATION

High blood sugar and high insulin levels combine to create inflammation in the body. Doctors define inflammation as a condition causing pain, swelling, redness, and heat. When you sprain your ankle or have an infected cut on your finger, you see the signs of inflammation. Your ankle swells up, hurts, gets red, and feels warm to the touch. The same thing happens to that cut on your finger. All this happens because your immune system is sending chemical signals and white blood cells to the area to heal the damage and fight the infection. When your ankle or finger heals, the inflammation goes away. That's good—your body is defending you against infection.

But what if the inflammation is caused by what you eat and how you live? Obesity, high blood sugar, smoking, lack of exercise, alcohol, lack of sleep, and poor diet all cause inflammation. If you're overweight, for example, fat could make up 25 percent or more of your body. Once you reach that level, your own fat becomes a source of inflammation.

By now, the inflammation is systemic—inside of you all over—instead of just in an injured place or because you're sick with something. The inflammation is now much less obvious, but it's still happening. It's a lot of the reason your back keeps hurting. If you're inflamed everywhere because of what you're eating, the process never stops, and you never heal. In fact, you get worse because the inflammation becomes chronic. Ongoing or chronic inflammation shows up as the underlying cause of a lot of other chronic health problems, including type 2 diabetes, heart disease, kidney disease, eye disease, autoimmune diseases, allergies, asthma, Alzheimer's disease, and even cancer. It also shows up as aching joints, back pain, skin problems, and frequent infections such as colds or cystitis.

High blood sugar also makes your red blood cells sticky and stiff. The sugar in your blood binds to the hemoglobin in the red blood cells and basically oxidizes it in a process called glycation. It's the same process that makes meat brown and sugar caramelize when cooking, except it's happening inside you. When your red blood cells are sticky and stiff, they don't circulate well into the capillaries, the tiniest blood vessels. In fact, they clog those vessels up, which is why people with diabetes are prone to damage to their retinas, their kidneys, their hearts, and their feet. Reduced capillary circulation happens all over the body, however. It's another reason your back hurts.

Cutting back on or eliminating flour also helps with gluten sensitivity. Some people have celiac disease, meaning they are seriously allergic to gluten, a protein found in wheat and other grains, including barley, rye, and oats. These people get severe intestinal inflammation and very unpleasant symptoms if they eat foods containing gluten. While true celiac disease is rare, being sensitive to gluten to a lesser degree turns out to be fairly common these days. It's possible that's because the wheat strains we eat today have been bred to be much higher in gluten than they were in earlier times.

Removing or reducing gluten in the diet seems to help some overweight people lose weight. This works well if you do it carefully. If you substitute high-carb, gluten-free products for wheat-containing foods, you're not accomplishing anything. Your blood sugar might even go higher and your inflammation level won't go down. The stores are full of products that are gluten-free but are still junk food. A gluten-free cookie isn't any better for you than one made with wheat flour.

The industrial oils we eat are also a problem. These are cheap vegetable oils made from corn, soybeans, canola, and other seeds that have been heavily processed and stripped of their nutrients. They're used in processed and prepared foods and as frying oil. They're everywhere in our diet—and they're a major source of inflammation. Industrial oils are so processed and unnatural that your body doesn't know what to do with them. When you eat these oils, which are high in omega-6 fatty acids, they make your cell membranes more rigid and make your arteries become thickened and stiff.

So not only can grains cause inflammation from increased

blood sugar and gluten, the oils in the grains add to the problem by causing arteriosclerosis, which can lead to high blood pressure and heart disease.

Chronic inflammation can be triggered by cellular dysfunction—when your cells aren't working right because of exposure to damaging free radicals, excess sugar in the blood, high levels of insulin, and other natural substances. The exposure damages the mitochondria, the tiny power plants within cells that convert glucose to energy.

INFLAMMATION AND PAIN

One of the hallmarks of inflammation is pain. That can be the pain of an inflamed area, like a sprained wrist, or it can be the pain of inflamed joints, or it can be more general aches and pains. But inflammation doesn't just cause pain, it makes you more sensitive to it. When you're inflamed internally, you're less resilient. Your body has a harder time making repairs to minor injuries. Your blood vessels are stiffer, and your blood doesn't circulate as well, so, when you're injured, your blood supply to the area isn't as efficient as it should be. Your ability to carry nutrients, white blood cells, and platelets to a damaged area—the muscles in your back, for instance—is restricted, so repairs don't happen as quickly. The discs in your spine have a relatively poor blood supply. They rely on the circulation around them for nutrients. If that circulation is poor, the discs are weakened; if they're damaged, they take longer to heal.

FAT FOR FUEL

If you don't eat anything white, then almost by definition, you're going to have a low-carbohydrate diet. You'll start feeling better and lose weight because now you're going to be using your own body fat as an energy source. You produce less insulin because you won't need as much to handle excess sugar in your system. Insulin also blocks your ability to burn fat as an energy source. The fat we carry around under our skin (subcutaneous fat) and in our abdomen (visceral fat) and in our liver is there to be used in times of need. If your body senses that you already have plenty of energy in the form of sugar, it says, "OK, lots of blood sugar right now. I don't need any more energy, so let's not burn that fat that's been building up." When you reduce the white processed foods in your diet, you start burning your stored fat instead. If you're already at a normal weight, you won't have to fight to stay there, because you'll be burning your calories before they become fat.

My patients get better when they stop eating white and processed foods. Their back pain becomes much more manageable even before they lose significant amounts of weight, they become more flexible, and their minor aches and pains get better. Of course, I'm not exactly the first doctor to notice that a low-carb diet is beneficial for my patients. The great Robert Atkins, M.D., pioneered the low-carb approach. His work has been built upon by others, such as William Davis, M.D., who wrote *Wheat Belly,* David Perlmutter, M.D., who wrote *Grain Brain,* and Dallas Hartwig and Melissa Hartwig, who wrote *The Whole30*. I strongly recommend these books to my patients so they can get a fuller picture of why cutting out white and processed foods is so important.

If the situation is serious and we can't wait for a patient to slim down a lot, I will operate on someone who is significantly overweight. I ask those patients to go on a very low-carb diet for three to four weeks or longer if possible before the surgery and to stay on it for at least three months afterward. Of course, I make sure they eat enough protein and enough good fats for good healing. They lose weight, but more importantly, their blood sugar level goes down, often dramatically. This really helps with healing after the surgery. Bad bacteria love sugar. If you don't feed it to them, your chances of a surgical infection drop and you also heal faster, with less discomfort.

GLUTEN SENSITIVITY

In medical school, we were taught about celiac disease, where some people are genetically severely intolerant of the gluten in grains. Starting in childhood (usually), these people get very ill with terrible gastrointestinal inflammation and often also arthritis-like symptoms. The only solution for people with celiac disease is to strictly avoid gluten in their diet.

What we've learned since my medical school days is that a lot more people than we realized have some degree of gluten intolerance. They don't get as sick as people with celiac disease, but they definitely can have symptoms that indicate their intestines don't like gluten. These people don't get the damaging level of intestinal inflammation that people with celiac disease get, but they still feel the effects of eating gluten. In particular, they feel joint and back pain.

Your digestion is a finely tuned machine for absorbing nutrients. It's entirely self-contained—the food you eat is absorbed from within it. If you're sensitive to gluten, however, the machine breaks down. Instead of absorbing nutrients correctly through the cells that line the intestines, the inflammation from gluten makes the tight junctions between those cells open up a bit. That lets molecules of undigested food enter the submucosal layer of the intestines. About 70 percent of the body's immune system cells are found in this part of the digestive tract, so when food particles end here, the body treats them as invaders. Inflammation is the result. Leaky gut syndrome, as this is called, pretty much goes away when you cut back on the amount of gluten you eat.

Leaky gut syndrome is the underlying cause of a lot of digestive problems and arthritic symptoms, along with other inflammation symptoms. It's possibly the underlying cause of a lot of autoimmune diseases, like multiple sclerosis and rheumatoid arthritis.

GLUTEN AND INFLAMMATION

I had a patient back in the late 1990s who had severely pinched nerves in her neck due to stenosis. She had severe arm pain. I operated on her to take the pressure off her nerves, and for a while, she felt better. Then her arms started hurting again. Even though now nothing was pressing on the cervical nerves in the area, they were very angry and inflamed. We couldn't find any mechanical reason. I had nothing but painkillers to offer. My patient decided to try something that she had heard about: she stopped eating gluten. When I saw her again for a three-month checkup, her arm pain had gone away. When she told me about the gluten, it didn't make sense to me, based on what I had been taught in medical school. But if it helped her, that was fine with me. I told her to keep doing what she was doing. I was intrigued by her success, to the point where I started looking into the research on gluten sensitivity. I read a lot of journal articles and learned that some nerves have gluten receptors in the myelin sheath that covers them. That made sense—and convinced me that there's much more to the role of inflammation than I had been taught in medical school.

INTERMITTENT FASTING

A lot of studies have shown that intermittent fasting can help reduce inflammation and improve overall health and energy. Intermittent fasting means eating all your normal calories, but within a shorter time frame of about eight to ten hours. This means you go about fourteen to sixteen hours without eating—from the time you finish your dinner until you have breakfast several hours after waking up. You would then have your normal lunch and dinner, but avoid eating after about 7 p.m.

Intermittent fasting makes your body use all the fuel you put into it, rather than storing some of it as fat. It's an especially effective technique if you also cut back on the carbs and processed foods. The theory behind intermittent fasting is that it aligns with what our bodies are adapted to. For most of human history, we were hunter-gatherers who didn't have a lot of extra food on hand and who went to sleep when it got dark, instead of staying up watching TV and eating snacks. Hunter-gatherers would normally eat most of their calories within a relatively short time frame. They would also sometimes go hungry when conditions were poor and sometimes have a lot of food when they were good. During the lean times, they would use their nutritional stores of fat. They used their calories efficiently, storing them as fat when they had extra but always needing to draw them down again long before a lot of fat accumulated. In our modern society, we never have lean periods where we need to burn our stored fat, even if we're normal weight. Intermittent fasting takes us back to a more natural eating pattern that helps prevent excess fat storage.

WEIGHT LOSS WITHOUT TRYING

One of the assistants in our office was normal weight and very fit, but when she got a new puppy, she lost weight. The new dog was very energetic and needed a lot of walking, especially first thing in the morning. My assistant found that she was skipping breakfast to take the dog out for a brisk two-mile walk. When she got home from that, the exercise had killed her appetite, plus she didn't have time for breakfast before she had to leave for work. She ended up coming in and having breakfast at her usual break time of 10 a.m. Then she had her lunch at her usual time of 12:30 p.m. When she got home at 6, she took the dog out again and ended up eating dinner at around 7. She usually didn't eat anything much after that and went to bed at her usual time.

Within a few months of this new routine, she was feeling great. She had lost a couple of pounds but also noticed that her clothes fit differently. They were looser around the waist. Her mildly arthritic right knee stopped hurting. She attributed it all to the extra exercise she was getting, but in fact, something else was going on: She was doing intermittent fasting without realizing it. All of her meals were now a bit larger than usual because the extra exercise made her a little hungrier. She still lost some weight in the abdominal area and felt great because she was compressing her calories into a shorter time frame. Instead of spreading them out between 7 a.m. and 7 p.m., she was eating them all between 10 a.m. and 7 p.m., and fasting for about twelve to fifteen hours. That was enough to make a difference in how well she metabolized her food and reduced the inflammation that was causing her knee pain.

At the cellular level, intermittent fasting may help slow aging. We know from animal studies that restricting calories keeps animals healthier and more active. They show fewer signs of aging, such as arthritis, than control animals who eat an unrestricted diet. The science behind is that caloric restriction affects the telomeres, the tips on the end of chromosomes that protect the genes—they're like the plastic tips on the ends of shoelaces. As we age, the telomeres get shorter, to the point where the chromosomes can't divide any longer, and the cell dies. Intermittent fasting seems to slow telomere shortening; the lab animals live longer and appear to be healthier. Intermittent fasting also promotes autophagy. At the cellular level, autophagy is a cleansing process that breaks down and recycles damaged molecules, misformed proteins, and cellular organelles. At the same time, intermittent fasting stimulates your body to produce growth hormones for making new cells and healing.

In humans, we know that intermittent fasting encourages safe, sustainable weight loss. It improves muscle mass and strengthens muscles, tendons, and ligaments. It lowers blood sugar spikes after meals. It also improves hemoglobin A1c, a measure of blood sugar over several months that's a good indicator of overall blood sugar levels and how well diabetes is controlled. It seems to help prevent or slow Alzheimer's disease and other forms of dementia. It may also help prevent cancer.

When your cells use glucose as fuel, the process creates a lot of free radicals or reactive electrons. You can think of free radicals as the exhaust from your car. You don't want to breathe it. Likewise, free radicals can do a lot of damage to your cells as they react with other cells. To deal with free radicals, your body has a wide range of antioxidant substances that latch onto them and stop them from doing damage. Your body has to make the antioxidants, however. If you're producing a lot of free radicals because of a diet high in carbohydrates, your antioxidant production might not be able to keep up. That means you have a lot more free radicals bouncing around your cells doing the sort of damage that leads to inflammation, arthritis, heart disease, and cancer. If you think of it in automotive terms, your engine is running too hot. Intermittent fasting cools things down by making you use glucose and fats for fuel much more efficiently.

CANCER PREVENTION

Cancer cells feed on glucose. Some studies suggest that if you don't have a lot of glucose in your system, cells that are just starting to become cancerous will die off from lack of food, instead of going on to grow larger and start dividing uncontrollably to cause cancer.

Based on the research findings about glucose, some researchers are now recommending going on a three- or four-day fast every quarter. The idea is that this will starve out precancerous cells because they can't survive without glucose. Similarly, going on a ketogenic (no carbs) diet during chemotherapy seems to lead to better outcomes.

VITAMIN D

Vitamin D is called a vitamin, but it's actually a hormone. It's a vitamin because it's something your body has to have but can't make enough for itself. You get most of your vitamins from the food you eat, but for vitamin D, you need to get sunshine on your skin. The sunshine starts the process that produces vitamin D inside your body.

You get some, but not a lot of vitamin D from your food, including fortified products such as milk. Most of the vitamin D in your body is manufactured in your kidneys in a complex process that begins with sunshine on your skin and ends with a hormone called calcitriol. Because your body makes calcitriol in one group of cells and sends it through the circulation to affect all the other cells in your body, it's a hormone. Among other things, calcitriol tells your bone cells what to do; it's essential for normal bone health. Without enough vitamin D, you're at risk for osteoporosis (thin, brittle bones that break easily) and osteopenia (thinning bones). I spend a lot of my time surgically repairing damage from thin bones. Vitamin D is also crucial for healthy collagen, an important part of cartilage and intervertebral discs—something else I spend a lot of time repairing.

If you're low on vitamin D, your bones and collagen won't be at optimal health. In my patients, that shows up as back and joint pain. When I test their blood for vitamin D levels, they're consistently too low. At least half of my back-pain patients are way below normal. Another quarter are somewhat below normal. Only about a quarter of them are in the normal range.

In fact, a lot of people are low on vitamin D because they don't get outdoors. Sunlight on your skin triggers the process that creates calcitriol, but you need to be outdoors in the sun for at least an hour a day for it to happen. We spend most of our time indoors, however, and we don't get much natural sunlight even in the summer. At the beach, we wear sunscreen, which blocks the UV light needed for vitamin D production. In the winter, the days are short and cold, and we spend as little time as possible with bare skin outdoors.

The RDA for vitamin D is between 600 and 800 IU a day. I feel this is far too low. Based on the research, I recommend 5,000 IU a day in the form of supplements to all my patients, even the ones who test in the normal range. The actual dose I recommend is individualized based on lab testing. The ones who are low start to feel better quickly. Interestingly, I see vitamin D help clinical depression in some patients. I tell those patients, "If you feel better, go talk to your doctor. Maybe you can stop your antidepressant medication."

Vitamin D supplements are very inexpensive and easy to find. Buy the supplements that contain vitamin D3, or cholecalciferol. This is the active form, which your body uses best. For cholecalciferol to work best, you also need adequate amounts of vitamin K. Leafy greens such as kale are the best dietary source of vitamin K. You can also take vitamin K supplements or take a combined vitamin D/K supplement. Vitamin K2 is another form of vitamin K, which may even be more important for Vitamin D metabolism. Vitamin K2 is found in many foods, including cheese, egg yolks, and butter.

STRENGTH TRAINING

Having strong muscles all over your body is important for preventing back pain. I have a patient who rides horses. His leg muscles are very strong, but he's having back pain. Why? Because the only muscles that are strong are in his legs. His arms aren't very toned at all. His other doctors had told him to stop riding, but my advice was to keep riding and add in weight training to strengthen his arms, shoulders, and abdominal muscles. When he started working on a weightlifting program with a trainer, his back pain disappeared.

One reason is that when you lift weights, you strengthen not only the muscles, but the bones and joints they're attached to. That helps spread the load across your back and takes some strain off the muscles that attach to the spine and the spine itself. When you move your joints while you lift weights, you move the fluid within the joint (synovial fluid), which carries more nutrients to and waste away from the cartilage and the capsule that surrounds the joint. Better nutrition helps keep joints healthy.

Lifting weights, moving, stretching, and strengthening all help with your structure and helps keep the spine in better alignment. If you have stronger core muscles and stronger arms, you have better posture and balance. Your spine isn't in an abnormal curve or angle that puts more stress at a particular joint or disc or bone, which can lead to early failure.

Lifting weights is ideal for keeping your back healthy because weight-bearing exercise helps to strengthen bones. You can do other exercises in addition to weight training. Yoga, Pilates, walking, biking, using an exercise bike or elliptical machine, swimming—anything that gets you moving all over is good. Just remember to do something weight-bearing if most of your exercise is coming from swimming, biking, or yoga, which don't put much stress on the bones.

Vibration machines are an interesting approach to bone strengthening. By just standing on a moving platform, your bones, muscles, and ligaments are stimulated, but doing exercises while on the platform has been shown to have even greater benefits. Vibration machines aren't an alternative to exercising, but they may be a good addition for people who can't exercise a lot because they have severe osteoporosis or some other limiting condition. Anecdotally, a lot of my patients and colleagues report good results.

INTERVAL TRAINING

Even before I was in medical school, I was very interested in fitness. I was browsing in the exercise physiology section of the library one day when I ran across a book about interval training—workouts that alternate periods of high-intensity exercise with low-intensity recovery periods—to improve fitness. That was revolutionary over thirty years ago. Today, interval training is widely used for improving fitness, especially heart health. Also known as high-intensity interval training (HIIT) or Tabata training, interval training is very easy to do. Every five to ten minutes during a workout, increase the intensity and do the exercise as hard as you can for just a minute or so. This works because anything that gets your heart rate up and lets it recover, then repeats the process several more times, builds up your endurance. Alternating exercise and recovery periods helps you get stronger, faster.

DON'T SMOKE

If you smoke, stop. You already know that smoking causes heart disease, stroke, and lung cancer, among other things. You may not know that smokers are at least three times more likely to have lower back pain. Only about 18 percent of the population smokes, but smokers make up about half of all people who seek pain treatment. Smoking makes arthritis and muscle pain worse.

The nicotine in tobacco is an addictive drug that has the

effect of increasing your sensitivity to pain. Nicotine constricts the smallest blood vessels and impairs the circulation of oxygen-rich blood to the body. By decreasing the amount of oxygen and nutrients that reach your tissues, bones, and joints, nicotine causes degeneration and osteoporosis. The discs in the spine don't have much circulation to begin with. Limiting the blood flow even more leads to a much greater likelihood of disc degeneration and rupture. Just one cigarette is enough to measurably affect blood flow. It takes at least four days for the effects of smoking on circulation to stop. Even if you quit smoking, your blood vessels will be constricted for at least four days afterward.

Tobacco breaks down collagen, which is why smokers not only get more arthritis but also get more facial wrinkles. Tobacco use also causes slower healing, both from collagen breakdown and from poor circulation. Any part of the body that's damaged hurts more and for longer. Even if you quit smoking, the part of your brain that deals with pain is still more sensitive for months afterward.

Tobacco use means that surgery to repair any sort of damage to the spine has a greater chance of failing. Also, you have a greater chance of developing an infection after the surgery. Smoking also raises the amount of carbon monoxide, a deadly poison, in your body. It takes at least 90 days to completely get rid of the carbon monoxide after your last cigarette. Like many other spine surgeons, I won't operate electively, unless it's an emergency, unless you have stopped smoking for at least eight weeks before the surgery and agree to stay away from tobacco for at least eight weeks, and preferably forever, after the surgery. To make sure you truly have stopped, I will test your blood for nicotine before the surgery, so don't try to cheat!

It's not easy to stop smoking, but help is readily available all around you. A good starting point is to call your local hospital to find out about free smoking cessation programs in your area. You can also call 1-800-QUIT-NOW for free help from trained coaches in your state. You may even qualify for free nicotine replacement patches to help you stop.

Doing all you can to help yourself heal your back pain is extremely important, but it may not be the complete answer. If you've lost weight, changed your diet, are exercising more, have stopped smoking, and done everything else you can and your back still hurts, it's time to investigate the causes. A precision diagnosis will help us decide on what your next steps should be.

CHAPTER 4

Precision Diagnosis

Russell had been having back pain ever since a car crash more than a decade ago. He'd seen doctors, physical therapists, chiropractors, and more doctors, but nobody could figure out where his pain was coming from. He'd had multiple X-rays and MRIs. None showed anything wrong. The pain was so severe that he was basically disabled, despite heavy narcotics doses.

I love treating patients like this because I love tracking down the source of this sort of problem and fixing it. Sometimes it's just a matter of going back to the basics and asking the right questions.

While Russell was telling me his story, I was watching how he sat. I could see he was subconsciously protecting the left side of his lower back in a way that took some pressure of his sacroiliac (SI) joint—the joint that connects the sacrum (the triangular bone at the bottom of the spine) with the pelvis. That told me he had an injury-causing instability in the SI joint, something that often doesn't show up on any imaging test. I asked him for more details about his accident, specifically if he "hit the brake" before the accident, and which foot he used. He drove like many race car drivers and jammed his left foot on the brake, and absorbing the impact up his leg to his lower back and SI joint. His story was so classic for this injury that I didn't need anything else to make the diagnosis. To be thorough, however, I needed confirmation.

I numbed the skin above the area and inserted a very thin needle directly into Russell's SI joint. I confirmed the needle was in place by injecting a little dye while I watched on a fluoroscope. Then I injected a small amount of a numbing medication into the joint, just like a dentist numbing a tooth before working on it. Russell felt almost immediate relief from the pain he had been feeling for many years, relief that lasted for the hour or so the numbing medicine worked.

That told me that Russell's car crash had created an instability in the joint that all his treatment so far hadn't diagnosed or helped. Braking with the left foot transferred the injury to his left SI joint. I later confirmed this even more precisely with an arthrogram, a test that uses X-rays or other imaging procedures and a contrast material to get very accurate images of a joint. The treatment was surgery to fuse the damaged, immobile joint. When Russell came back two weeks later for a checkup, he was off all narcotics and had only normal, very manageable post-op pain.

IMAGING FOR DIAGNOSIS

The precision of the needle diagnosis helped pinpoint Russell's problem when other techniques had failed. That's not to say X-rays, MRIs, and other imaging approaches don't help, because in many cases they help enormously. I use imaging all the time as part of the overall workup and evaluation—the images are part of the bigger picture.

For patients with sciatica that keeps coming back, for instance, an MRI will show me if there's a disc herniation that's pinching the nerve. That's something I can't tell just from a patient's history and a physical exam. It will also tell me if other discs around the herniated one are also herniated or bulging. Once I can see the herniation, then I have a real target to aim for in the surgery. I only need a small incision of a couple of centimeters to get down to where that damaged disc is and move the bulging piece off the nerve. Taking out a small piece of the disc herniation that's annoying your nerve is like being able to reach inside your shoe and take out a small pebble that's annoying you.

X-RAYS

The simplest imaging test is the X-ray, something doctors have been using since the early 1900s. X-rays can only show us the bones, not any soft tissue such as ligaments, tendons, or muscles. We can infer where soft tissue like discs are because there's a space in between the vertebrae that shows up as a space between the bones.

X-rays can be helpful for showing a fracture or something that's severely displaced. For sciatica and other types of back pain, the X-ray is much more useful if it's taken while you're standing up so I can see how the spine is aligned relative to gravity. If you're lying down, the X-ray doesn't give me all the information available. I want the image to show your spine from the front and also from the side while you're standing upright.

Gravity will show me that a disc is collapsed, leaving no space between the vertebrae. The same space might open up, however, when you're lying down. Gravity may also show that the spine is no longer aligned correctly because you have some instability.

A plain X-ray just while you're standing up may not show much. When you bend forward or backward at the hips, however, that often shows the damaged area, because your spine has a little bit of give at every disc. If there's an injury to a disc, it may show motion when you're bending that doesn't show up when you're lying down or standing upright. Those images are important clues for finding instability.

FLUOROSCOPY

A fluoroscope is a machine that shows a continuous X-ray image on a monitor. It's like looking at an X-ray movie. In the exam room, fluoroscopy lets me see how your spine moves in real-time and lets me snap a series of X-ray pictures as you move. In the procedure room or operating room, fluoroscopy lets me see where my instruments are instead of guessing based on anatomical landmarks. It lets me be very precise. Fluoroscopy allows me to put skinny needles down to specific joints or near a specific nerve to precisely place medicine where it is needed.

ULTRASOUND

Ultrasound is another technique used to see things non-invasively within the body. It is usually used to image soft tissues and can be helpful in directing injections or other minimally invasive procedures as well.

You may be familiar with seeing ultrasound pictures of babies in a mother's womb. The ultrasound can be used to see other things, like muscle and tendon tears, to evaluate cysts and bumps, and other things like this.

CT SCAN

A CT scan is basically a very elaborate X-ray using computerized tomography to take a lot of pictures in slices through your body and then put them together into one or a series of images. While you're having the CT, we sometimes inject you with a small amount of contrast material to make the soft tissue and nerve details show up better. A CT also shows shadows of soft tissue like muscle.

CT scans are great for people who have pacemakers or other internal hardware that means they can't have an MRI. They're also great for seeing how well you're healing from a broken bone. With a CT scan, I can see small fractures or cracks that might not show up on an X-ray. CT scans are good for looking at vertebrae fusions, especially to see any areas that didn't fuse properly from previous surgery. I can also see any hardware, such as screws, that remain in your spine from previous surgery. Those don't show up well in an MRI at all.

For diagnosing back pain, I often want to see both X-rays and CT scans. Some patients object to this because they don't want any extra radiation exposure. That's a good point, and it's a good reason to be cautious about too much testing. Most of the exposure comes from the CT, however, not the X-ray. I need both because the CT has to be done while you're lying down. That affects the way the discs appear and can make them falsely look normal. The X-rays give me the additional information I need to see how your spine looks dynamically, not just when lying down.

MRIS

For the most detailed look at the spine and the soft tissue around it, the MRI is by far the best test. X-rays are the quickest, easiest, and cheapest way to image the spine. If the problem is just in the bones, like a fracture, X-rays are great. But for more detail that shows the soft tissue as well, MRIs are the best. The MRI uses magnetism, not radiation, to create the image. It takes much longer, it's very noisy, it's expensive, and it's nowhere near as convenient as an X-ray, but it shows me more of what I need to see in great detail. An MRI shows not just the bones but also the soft tissue, the nerves, and even the fat in the area.

An MRI can show an area of infection or a tumor in the spine that I can't see otherwise. I can see the discs themselves because collagen shows up. I can also see the outlines of nerves, which lets me see exactly which ones are being pinched.

Usually, I order both an X-ray and an MRI, which will allow me to assess the boney alignment and stability (X-ray), as well as the soft tissue, discs, and nerves (MRI). These tests are complementary, and together are very useful.

BONE SCAN

A bone scan is another way to image the spine and look for the source of unexplained lower back pain. For this test, a tiny amount of a radioactive substance called a tracer is injected into a vein. The tracer travels around your body and gets picked up by your bones. A special camera then takes pictures of the bones in question. The parts of the bones that don't absorb any or just a little tracer show up as dark spots, often called cold spots. A cold spot tells me that the blood supply to that area is restricted. When a bright spot, also called a hot spot, shows up, that indicates an area of increased blood flow. A hot spot tells me the area has an area of fast bone repair, arthritis, or an infection, or maybe a fracture or tumor.

The nuclear bone scan is a very sensitive test. We'll often see stress fractures that don't show up on CT scans well or take a few days before they show up on an X-ray or MRI. We can see things early, like little cracks in the spine that indicate areas of inflammation that can warn of impending injury, such as a stress fracture. The bone scan can give me a clue that the area is still trying to heal. It can also help diagnose infection, ligament injury, or bruises, which can be a hard-to-find cause of back pain.

ARTHROGRAM

An arthrogram is an imaging test used to look inside a joint, such as your hip or shoulder, and get a good view of the cartilage, tendons, and ligaments. A contrast material such as a dye is injected into the joint or into your bloodstream. The joint is then imaged using X-rays, CT scans, or an MRI to get a series of pictures.

MYELOGRAM

We use myelograms to look at the spinal canal to see if that's the source of your back pain. During the test, a dye (or "contrast") is injected into the space of the spinal canal. We then use X-rays or a CT scan to see if there's any nerve compression caused by a herniated disc or a fracture. If there's a disc herniation, the bulging part pushes into that space. I can see it because it displaced the dye from the outside. This is a good test for people who can't be exposed to the magnetism of the MRI machine because they have a pacemaker. It's a little more complicated than other tests, however. You may need to go to a hospital or specialized imaging center to have it done by a specialist in interventional radiology.

DISCOGRAPHY

A myelogram, which injects dye around nerves, isn't the same as a discography, which is a test that uses dye or saline injected right into a disc. We don't do this too often because it can be painful, but if we're having trouble figuring out where the pain is coming from, it's a good way to learn if the problem is in a particular disc. We use it when someone has a lot of back pain that's made worse by prolonged sitting or when we've tried all sorts of other nonsurgical treatments and none of it has helped. We're trying to find out if the pain is caused by the disc itself, not by the disc pressing on a nerve as it does when it's herniated. We use a very thin needle to go right into the jelly-like center of the disc itself and inject a small amount of dye or saline solution. Typically, right after the injection, the patient says, "I can feel something, a little pressure there." Sometimes, though, the patient says, "Wow, you found it," or "You just kicked me there, right?" That's when the liquid has irritated the damaged disc, which definitely hurts.

Discography lets us see if the disc is contributing to the pain. More importantly, it lets us see which discs aren't involved so we can narrow it down to the right place and be sure that there's no other reason for the symptoms.

SCOLIOSIS IMAGING

Patients who have scoliosis, or too much side-to-side curve in their spine, need special imaging to help me see the whole alignment of the spine. When you stand upright, your head should be balanced over your pelvis and your knees. That's the most efficient way to stand. If you have scoliosis, you can't stand upright well—you're always working hard to balance yourself, which can lead to a lot of pain and disability. If the curve gets big enough, it starts constricting the space for the heart and lungs so much that they can't work well.

Scoliosis imaging helps us measure balance for people with scoliosis and see if it's balancing out over time, as sometimes happens with adolescents, or if it's progressing. If we see it progressing over time, surgery might be needed.

Instead of the very precise scoliosis X-rays, we can use the EOS system. This is a new system that's very expensive, so it's not that common yet in smaller hospitals. EOS is a 3-D imaging system that uses X-rays to show the spine in great detail while you're standing upright. It's very valuable for diagnosing scoliosis and planning treatment. Scoliosis is mostly a problem in kids and teenagers. They need a lot of imaging at a time when they're also growing fast, which means they're more vulnerable to radiation damage. The images in EOS are done with very low dose X-rays, which are much safer for these patients.

IMAGING ISSUES

Modern technology lets us get very accurate looks at the spine and the surrounding tissue. The imaging doesn't always tell the whole story, though, especially soon after an injury.

When you're injured or have an infection, your body has an inflammatory response and sends white blood cells and other natural chemicals to the area. That can take a few days to be visible on an X-ray or MRI. So, you might have an MRI today because you were in an accident and your back hurts, but the damage might not show up. A compression fracture, for example, will take a few days or even a week to become visible. I've had patients with compression fractures who looked perfectly normal on an X-ray soon after it happened. They come back three weeks later because their back still hurts. At that point, I can see that the bone has now collapsed by 50 percent because it was so weakened by the fracture. That's why I have them do repeat X-rays a few days after the accident. I also frequently do repeat X-rays in the office every six months when I'm following someone for a problem. The X-ray from three years ago just isn't good enough anymore.

If you have an infection, it might not show up right away, but six weeks later, a disc might be destroyed because the infection was there long enough to do real damage. Sometimes we need to do a series of images to try to catch something.

OPERATING ROOM IMAGES

When I'm doing surgery, I have the patient's most recent MRIs and X-rays up on a monitor. At the start of the surgery, I'll take another X-ray of the area using radio-opaque markers as a guide to where to get into the spine area. Once I get down to the spine, I put another marker there and take another picture to confirm I'm in the right place. I can also bring in a portable CT machine, called an O-arm, to take more images with registration marks attached to the spine. Sometimes I can even use computer-generated virtual reality (VR) imaging. I use all the imaging to see where my instruments are and make sure I'm hitting exactly the part of the bone I want to reach. I also have an electrical neuromonitoring device that sends me a signal if I get too close to a nerve. All this live monitoring makes the surgery very cool stuff, plus it makes the surgery that much safer and accurate.

Modern imaging is used for diagnosis and in surgery, but it's also used in some nonoperative treatments for relieving back pain. That's where we're going with the next chapter.

CHAPTER 5

Nonoperative Treatments

Women's roller derby isn't the dangerous sport it used to be, but it's still rough on the body. The women wear helmets and elbow and knee pads, but these few pads don't protect all of your body when you fall. In particular, they don't protect your buttocks. When Kathleen (or Killer, as she's known to her teammates and fans), took a spill during a roller derby competition, she landed hard on her bottom, enough to cause a small wedge fracture in her spine.

That's a painful injury. When I examined Kathleen, I saw she didn't need surgery to decompress anything and recommended a brace instead. She wore the brace for a few weeks, but it wasn't helping. I ended up stabilizing the fracture by inserting a small needle into the bone and putting in some bone cement. It was like putting a cast inside the bone. She felt better within 10 minutes, the time it took for the cement to harden.

Bone cement is a good example of how we can treat a lot of back pain without surgery. The list of effective, nonoperative treatments is long.

INJECTIONS

My first choice of a nonoperative therapy if time, physical therapy, and other treatments aren't working, is often an injection. The injection is typically a numbing medicine, sometimes along with steroids, into the painful area. This often relieves back or neck pain enough so that the area has a chance to heal on its own. Typically, I use a combination of a numbing medication such as lidocaine or Marcaine along with a small dose of a corticosteroid such as methylprednisone. The numbing medicine often gives immediate pain relief. The steroid is a powerful anti-inflammatory drug that brings down the swelling around the nerve, which is often the cause of the pain. The steroid usually kicks in by the next day or two and calms the inflammation. Sometimes that's enough to cure the problem. More often, the pain is under control for a month or two, which is long enough to do some physical therapy to stabilize the area. Injecting the steroid instead of taking pills is like the difference between putting ice on where it hurts and drinking iced tea. The injections work directly on the painful area.

Alternatively, the injection can be with PRP—platelet-rich plasma—which also has anti-inflammatory properties. There are a host of other healing factors that are also either within PRP or are stimulated by PRP, which can promote healing.

My patients often ask, "Is this injection going to cure me?" I can only say, "It depends." If the damage isn't that bad, the injection will probably help quite a bit and may even cure the problem. But if it's more serious, the injection will just calm the nerves down for a short time, relieve your discomfort, and give you a chance to heal.

Injections into the spine are usually guided by fluoroscopy or ultrasound. When I train pain management doctors on how to do injections, they frequently think they already know how, because they use injections into muscles all the time. They quickly realize that the spine needs special techniques for knowing where to do the injection and, crucially, knowing when you're in the right spot. I teach them how to visualize the anatomy and then use the fluoroscope or ultrasound to guide where the tip of the needle goes.

Injections can also be used to diagnose the real problem. I'll often see someone with both neck pain and shoulder pain. Is the pain coming primarily from a pinched nerve in the neck and radiating into the shoulder? Or is it coming from bursitis or a rotator cuff tear in the shoulder that's also making the neck hurt? One good way to find out is to do a subacromial injection of lidocaine and a steroid—that's an injection right above the shoulder joint, where the bursa (the fluid-filled sac that lets the joint move smoothly) is. I give the medicine about thirty seconds to work and then ask them to raise their arm above their head. If they can now do that easily with no pain, that tells me the source of the pain is bursitis or a small rotator cuff tear in the shoulder. If the shot doesn't make any difference, that tells me the pain is more likely from a pinched nerve in the neck.

Injections also help me figure out the exact source of the pain. We can't see "pain" on imaging studies. Sometimes we see things that look like they should hurt, but they don't. We also see things that look perfectly normal but hurt a lot. If we inject numbing medication into an area and it helps, that gives us a clue about whether we have the right place or not.

Because injections are partially therapeutic and partially diagnostic, I ask my patients to keep a pain log daily for three or four weeks after the injection. When I see them again for a follow-up and ask them how the injection went, they often say, "It didn't work." When we go through their log, though, it reminds them that it did help initially. They say, "You know, for the first two days I felt great and then the pain slowly came back." By helping them remember the full story and how their pain changed over time, we get the full diagnostic benefit.

The problem with injections is that they're not that predictable. Sometimes the benefit lasts for months, sometimes for much less time. We often don't know if it's going to last until we do it. I recently had a patient who told me he had tried injections years ago without success. He ended up having surgery for a disc herniation. It helped, but now, eight years later, he was in my office with back pain again. Nothing else was working, so before we went to the surgical option, I suggested trying an injection. He was reluctant at first because of his previous experience, but I told him, "Well, last time is last time. Things have changed. This time might be different." Before, the problem was a pinched nerve. I felt that this time, because he'd had surgery for the pinched nerve, the problem was more likely to be inflammation. It was. He came back two weeks later and told me he was completely pain-free. Why did it work this time and not before? Hard to say for sure, but it's possible that this time around he didn't have a herniated disc, just something mildly irritating that the injection was able to calm down. The important thing is he was feeling much better and was back to leading a normal, active life.

I'll sometimes try a dose pack of an oral steroid drug such as methylprednisolone (Medrol) before going to an injection. Prednisone can be a good choice for short-term treatment, but it's a powerful drug. When it's taken orally, it affects your whole system, not just your injured back, so it has to be used cautiously. The dose pack is designed to taper down the dosage over a week or ten days.

As I mentioned before, sometimes instead of injecting steroids, other things can be used—such as PRP, PPP, stem cells, fibrinogen, and other biologics, to name a few. Each has its reason and purpose. It's important to be able to have a lot of options and tools available in order to try to decrease someone's pain. Even more options follow.

IDET

Intradiscal electrothermal annuloplasty (IDET) is a minimally invasive treatment for chronic lower back pain caused by some kinds of disc damage. I use it when the disc itself is the problem—not when the disc is pressing on a nerve.

We know that most back pain will get better in three to six months without surgery. If you're still in pain after six months, however, the situation changes. We need to look more closely at your spine, and specifically, we need to look at your discs. Sometimes the disc isn't herniated; it's injured. As I explained in chapter 2, the discs between your vertebrae are shock absorbers like jelly donuts, with a tough outer covering and a squishy, jelly-like center. The center doesn't have any nerves, but the outer covering does. An injured disc is going to make your back hurt because it's injured, not because it's been squished out of shape and is now pressing on a nerve.

To see if disc injury is the cause of your pain, I'll do a discogram. If that shows the disc is damaged and painful, I can do an IDET procedure to relieve the pain. Disc injury, as opposed to a herniated disc pressing on a nerve, isn't that common. That means I don't use this procedure very often, but when I do, it really works well.

IDET uses heat at 90° C (194° F) delivered slowly through a catheter directly to the damaged disc for up to twenty minutes. The heat makes the disc thicken and shrink, which relieves the pain. It works something like this: Imagine if you were to take a strand of your hair, which is made of collagen, and hold it against the heat of an incandescent light bulb, you'll see it shrink up. That's very similar to what I'm doing to a damaged disc with IDET. When the disc shrinks, tiny tears in it are sealed up. It's also possible that the heat destroys the pain receptors inside the disc. To be honest, we don't know for sure why this procedure works so well on the right patient, but it does. IDET is usually done on an outpatient basis without an overnight hospital stay. The procedure takes about an hour and needs only a small incision in the skin. Most patients feel a lot better within a few weeks, although complete healing can take up to six months.

When I do this for my patients, the benefit lasts for at least a couple of years. At least half can postpone disc fusion surgery, which gives them a chance to lose weight if they need to, or even avoid surgery completely. I've had some patients feel good for ten years before needing further treatment.

When IDET first became available in 1997, a lot of pain doctors jumped on it as a miracle cure. I think it was used too often on people whose pain wasn't severe enough or wasn't applied to the right patient. Some of the doctors who did it were making a lot of money but weren't helping their patients that much. Then we had a very small double-blind study that supposedly showed IDET didn't make much difference, even though many patients have had good relief. That gave insurers a reason to stop paying for it, even though IDET is FDA approved. It may have been used far too often when it first came out, but for the patient whose back pain can be traced to one or two discs that aren't worn out yet, it can be a good treatment.

BASIVERTEBRAL NERVE ABLATION

The basivertebral nerve (BVN) is a nerve that innervates the endplates of the vertebral bodies of the spine. It innervates the part of the vertebra that supports the discs of the spine.

What is so special about this nerve?

There are nerves that sense pain in the facet joints (the joints in the back of the spine), nerves that innervate the discs themselves (this is what happens when discs themselves are injured or hurt, which is why a discography test is often used), and there are nerves that innervate the endplates of the vertebral bodies above and below the disc, where the disc sits. These endplate nerves are the BVNs.

Very recently, a new procedure has been made available, and is FDA approved for vertebrogenic low back pain—the pain caused by inflammation of or damage to the vertebral endplates and sensed by the BVN.

This minimally invasive procedure, which has been studied for over ten years and has over five-year outcomes in a well-designed, double-blind clinical study, is recently being made available. The procedure is a nerve ablation of the BVN, similar to a facet rhizotomy, but performed on the nerve within the vertebral body, which is where the BVN is.

This outpatient, percutaneous procedure is demonstrating very good outcomes that are long-lasting. And it is currently only available from specially trained surgeons in order to keep the quality of outcomes high. The registered brand for this procedure is the "Intracept" procedure.

Again, as mentioned previously, it is important to have a precise diagnosis in order to have the best potential outcomes for any procedure. Doing this precise procedure in an attempt to treat just any cause of low back pain won't work. However, for the carefully selected, correct patient, it has helped many people decrease or eliminate their chronic back pain.

REGENERATIVE MEDICINE

Regenerative medicine techniques such as stem cells, prolotherapy, and platelet-rich plasma can all be helpful for back pain. I'll discuss those cutting-edge techniques in chapter 6.

RHIZOTOMY

Rhizotomy, also called radiofrequency denervation or nerve ablation, is another technique that uses heat, but directly to the nerves, not the disc. The procedure is sometimes done to relieve back pain caused by damage to the facet joint in the lower back or to relieve pain caused by the sacroiliac joint. The most common reason for doing it is when injections have helped, but only for a short time. That tells us that numbing the nerve in the painful area helps, but we need to do it in a more long-lasting way. That's where rhizotomy comes in. With this technique, we can numb the small pain fibers in the area for much longer, usually from six months to a year or even longer. After that, the small pain nerves grow back. In the meantime, though, you're now able to work on the problem in other ways, such as lifestyle changes and physical therapy, so the pain may not come back.

To do a rhizotomy, I numb the area and then insert a needle into it. I already have a good idea of where the pain is coming from, but to find exactly where the painful small nerves are, I put a little electrical stimulation through the needle. I'll ask as I do it, "Where do you feel this?" When you tell me that I've found the spot where you feel the pain, I then apply radiofrequency stimulation to the needle. That's basically heat, which very gently burns the nerve fiber and makes it stop working. I'm creating a lesion on a nerve that's the thickness of a hair, so the procedure is quite safe.

This procedure can also be done using endoscopy. An endoscope is a camera, and it can be used to go and actually look at the small nerves near the facet joints. Using this camera, I can see directly where these small nerves are, and they can be directly cut or heated. Since a larger area is able to be directly seen, this method may last even longer than the percutaneous method. However, both techniques usually work quite well.

EXERCISE

Exercise to strengthen the core muscles of the body is extremely helpful for people with back pain. (I'll discuss physical therapy, which is guided exercise for dealing with a specific problem at the end of this chapter.) Your core is made up of the muscles that hold you upright, including your abdominal muscles, your back muscles, and the muscles around the pelvis, including your buttocks. If your core is strong, it forms a strong link between your lower body and your upper body and head. Strong core muscles make it easier to do the activities of daily living, like carrying in groceries from the car and picking up a child. A strong core helps prevent back strains and improves your posture.

You can build up your core muscles just by doing simple exercises at home, like squats and planks. You need to do these exercises most days for them to help your back, so if you can't get to a gym that often, work with a trainer to get started and ask them to teach you a manageable home routine.

The human body is designed to move. Unfortunately, most of us spend most of our time not moving—we sit instead. That's bad for your health in general and particularly bad for your back. I strongly advise all my patients to move as much as possible. I tell them, "Sitting is the new smoking. Don't do it." Anything that gets you up and moving will help. If at all possible, don't sit for more than thirty minutes at a time. Get up and walk around or at least do some stretching for a few minutes. A lot of sitting happens while watching TV. That's a great opportunity to enjoy your show while you ride an exercise bike, do yoga, stretch, lift weights, or do anything else that gets you moving.

PILATES

Pilates is an exercise system that uses low-impact exercises and stretches to strengthen the core muscles and improve flexibility and balance. The system was developed by Joseph Pilates, a fitness instructor who developed the basic concepts during World War I. His system was embraced by dancers and other performers starting in the 1920s. It's since become more popular with the general public as a great way to build core strength and stability. Pilates can be particularly helpful for back pain.

One of my physician assistants decided to become a Pilates instructor, so I've taken a lot of Pilates classes at her studio. Studio Pilates uses some specialized equipment that's not designed for home use, but you can also do a lot of Pilates exercises at home with just a mat and some very minimal, inexpensive equipment. I recommend Pilates to my patients frequently. Most report good results, but like any exercise, it only helps if you stick with it. Again, work with a certified Pilates instructor to learn the basics safely and design a regular home routine.

YOGA

In 2017, an important study in *Annals of Internal Medicine,* published by the American College of Physicians, compared yoga with standard physical therapy for treating chronic lower back pain. The study showed that yoga was as effective as physical therapy for relieving pain and reducing the use of pain medication. That result didn't surprise me, because I had already seen similar positive benefits in myself and in my patients who did yoga.

I recommend yoga to a lot of my patients. In fact, I think it's so valuable that I'm a certified yoga instructor. Yoga comes in a number of different styles. I find that the more active Vinyasa style, which is fairly athletic but still gentle, is particularly good for my back pain patients. It helps them become more flexible and improves their balance. Because you hold positions, it also strengthens the arms, legs, and core.

The only restriction on yoga I have is for my patients with neck pain or neck injuries. I don't want them doing headstands or shoulder stands. Of course, if any position is painful, stop doing it. A good yoga instructor will help you modify the positions to do them safely.

Yoga class can be very relaxing and it's fun to learn new positions. If you can't make it to a class regularly, go at least a few times to get a good grasp of the basics. You can then easily do yoga at home.

WEIGHT TRAINING

Weight training, also called resistance training, can be very helpful for improving back pain. It's an efficient, safe way to build muscle strength and improve stability and posture. As an added plus, it's literally a weight-bearing exercise, which builds bone and helps protect you from osteoporosis. For many of my patients, the best thing about weight training is the way it builds their overall strength, which helps a lot of with the activities of daily living. If you're stronger, you can manage chores like vacuuming and carrying laundry baskets much more easily.

The key to weight training without injury is to have good form. You want to stimulate muscle growth and build strength without over-lifting or lifting the wrong way. Work with a trainer to get started off correctly with good form and the right set of exercises. Be very careful not to do too much, too fast, too soon.

Another key item is to do the exercises under control, and not to "throw" the weights around. A very good technique is to lift and lower the weights slowly and in a controlled fashion for ten to fifteen seconds each rep. This super slow technique can help stimulate muscles while protecting the underlying joint and tendon. This is a key item for everyone, especially the elderly.

BETTER NUTRITION

I've already discussed nutrition in chapter 3, but it's so important as a way to avoid back surgery that I want to bring it up again in this chapter as well. I truly see making changes in what you eat as a form of nonoperative treatment for back pain. This goes beyond the reality that being overweight is a big factor in causing back pain and losing weight helps.

The standard American diet (SAD) is far too high in sugar and processed carbohydrates. SAD is badly imbalanced in the types of dietary fats it includes. This diet is a prescription for inflammation—and inflammation is the root cause of most severe back pain. Inflammation predisposes you to back injury, it makes the pain worse, and it makes the injury take longer to heal.

I ask my patients to get back to the basics of a healthy diet. I ask them to give up the sugary foods, the high-calorie, low-nutrition junk foods, and the fast foods laden with bad fats. I ask them to eat less processed food and a lot more vegetables and greens. I ask them to shift the balance of their dietary fat to a healthier ratio. I also ask my patients to make sure they get adequate protein in their diet.

The RDA for protein—the amount you need for basic health—is about 0.4 grams per pound of body weight, or about 10 percent of your daily calories. For example, if you're a sedentary person who weighs 150 pounds, you need to get at least 54 grams of protein a day. To put that in perspective, there are 7 grams of protein in an ounce of cheddar cheese, a chicken leg has 13 grams, and a six-ounce steak has 42 grams.

I think the RDA is too low for optimal health, particularly if you're fairly active or are over age forty-five, when you start to need more protein to help maintain muscle mass and strong bones. Remember, the RDA is designed for a healthy person to avoid disease, and is the minimum among suggested. I suggest aiming for a minimum of 1 gram of protein for every pound of lean body weight. To get that protein, aim for foods that are also good sources of omega-3 fatty acids, such as fish, eggs, pastured beef and poultry, and nuts.

More recent studies are suggesting slightly higher amounts of protein per day, since protein is essential for many functions in the body. At this time, a minimum of 1 gram per pound of body weight per day is recommended, and possibly more if exercising, healing, or preparing for surgery. Again, more recent studies suggest that we should have even more—1.6 to 2.2 grams of protein/kilogram/day. That is 1 gram per pound! Protein is needed for muscle and for bone, and healing, especially if we are undergoing stress like surgery, exercise, or healing. Some studies suggest that the majority of people undergoing surgery are under- or malnourished, so they need this. Further, studies show that protein does not increase cancer risks, nor affect the kidneys (despite what many of us were originally taught.) As we age, we need more protein as well. These are important factors to account for in your diet.

SUPPLEMENTS

A lot of back pain comes from osteoarthritis in the spine. The supplements glucosamine and chondroitin sulfate are often recommended for helping joint pain from arthritis. The evidence for these supplements helping knee and hip pain is fairly strong—if you happen to be a strong responder. About a third of the people who try these supplements, which are usually combined together, do get good pain relief. Another third get some benefit, but a third don't. The evidence that these supplements help back pain from osteoarthritis is less compelling. They're worth trying—they might help and they're unlikely to harm.

Additional collagen may be more valuable for back pain. Your discs are made mostly of collagen, the most abundant protein in the body, so getting some extra in your diet may help them heal. You can try having bone broth every day—this is just soup made from beef or chicken bones flavored with vegetables and simmered for a long time to get the collagen out of the bones. You can make your own (lots of recipes online) or buy it fresh or frozen. You can also just take supplements.

Protein, vitamins, and minerals can also be supplemented.

Ideally, these macro and micronutrients would be readily bioavailable in regular foods, but this is often not the case. It is important to source and choose your foods well, and to eat whole foods. New recommendations in the field of immunonutrition provide significant improvements in postoperative healing as well as in overall health. It is important to stay up-to-date with these advances. The specifics of supplementation should be individualized and discussed with a well-trained provider.

HEAT

Sometimes a simple heating pad is all you need to relax the muscles around your spine. You can also try infrared heat, which can help with muscle spasms and fatigue. Infrared heat lamps are inexpensive and easy to find. They're not the magic cure some claim them to be, but the warmth can be very soothing. Infrared heat can help the muscles and blood vessels relax in order to increase blood flow to the area. The increased blood flow can aid in healing.

Also, some infrared lights serve to stimulate mitochondria, the energy houses of the cell. More robust and healthy mitochondria are essential for good health. Both the heat and the light provided by infrared sources can be useful in treating muscles and back pain.

ACUPUNCTURE AND DRY NEEDLING

Acupuncture for acute and chronic back pain has been extensively studied for years. The evidence that it works is fairly strong. In fact, it's good enough that the Agency for Healthcare Research and Quality (AHRQ) recommended it in a 2016 review article of noninvasive treatments for chronic low back pain.

There's certainly something to be said for a treatment that's been around for some 2,500 years. Acupuncture uses very thin needles inserted just a little way into the skin along meridians, or energy pathways. The needles stimulate the points and improve the flow of energy. There are more scientific explanations for why it works, but the point is that in skilled hands, acupuncture can be useful for relieving back pain. The treatment relieves the pain enough so that the body's natural healing strength can take over.

Years ago, you had to search out an acupuncture therapist who had been trained in China, but today a lot of practitioners, including medical doctors, are licensed to do acupuncture safely and effectively. If one of my patients wants to try it, I encourage them to go ahead. Most of my patients who have been helped by acupuncture needed about ten weekly sessions.

Dry needling is similar to acupuncture, but it's more for helping a spasming muscle relax. A very thin acupuncture needle is inserted right into the trigger point to stop the spasm. The needle stops the feedback loop of pain-spasm-pain-spasm. A lot of emergency room doctors and nurses use it to treat people who come in with severe back, neck, or shoulder pain. Studies have shown that dry needling can relieve the immediate pain of a muscle spasm and can also help a patient break through an impasse in the healing process.

I've had a lot of patients who reached a plateau with other treatments. Their pain was better, but still bad. After anywhere from four to twelve dry needling sessions, they're usually able to get past the muscle spasms and achieve measurably improved pain scores and better range of motion. When they're not in as much pain, they can do more stretching and exercise. That lets them move off the pain plateau and start the healing journey again.

For both acupuncture and dry needling, the needles are sterile and are used just once. They're very, very skinny. You don't feel them going in and they don't leave a bruise or mark. If you did feel them going in at all, it's just a tiny prick.

BRACING

Bracing can be very useful for neck pain. If you're having numbness in your hands, for instance, using a neck brace can help us figure out if the numbness is coming from a pinched nerve in the cervical vertebrae or from some other problem, like carpal tunnel syndrome. If the neck brace helps, it's the vertebrae. If wrist braces help, it's carpal tunnel. A neck brace can also be helpful if you have a painful neck sprain or strain. Wearing either a soft or more rigid collar for a few days can help with the pain and give those neck muscles a rest. Wearing the brace any longer than that can lead to muscle atrophy. You lose muscle strength and start becoming reliant on the collar. The collar is to get you past the worst of the pain so we can get you into physical therapy.

For lower back pain, bracing can be helpful for people who have some slight instability in their sacroiliac joints. Wearing a brace that's similar to a weightlifting belt can help stabilize the area and improve the pain. Compression-type braces can sometimes be helpful for calming down local inflammation in the lower back and lumbar region, but they should only be used for a short time. Again, we don't want the muscles in the area to get weaker. The brace is just to relieve the pain enough so you can start physical therapy to get those muscles stronger.

SPINAL CORD STIMULATION

Some pain specialists prescribe spinal cord stimulators to relieve back pain. I've been using them for years—long before the pain doctors in my area started using them as well. The theory is that if someone has a really damaged spinal nerve, even if nothing is pinching it anymore, it still hurts. The nerve is just stuck in pain-signaling mode—and your brain may be stuck in pain-receiving mode. If the nerve is stimulated by something that doesn't cause pain, it can reduce or even nullify the pain signal, because only one stimulation can go through the gate at a time. When a non-stimulus fills the gate, it blocks anything else from going through it, and it keeps out the pain stimulus.

This is called the gate control theory of pain. The idea is that pain depends on your response to the interplay between your central nervous system (the brain and spinal cord) and your peripheral nervous system (all the other nerves, including the ones in your lower back). When you injure your back, the pain sensation flows from your peripheral nerves to your central nervous system and up to the brain. A stimulator works to interrupt this pain pathway from the extremity to the brain. The stimulator adds a different sensation to the pathway, which closes the gate to the brain.

The gate control theory says that the spinal cord has "nerve gates" that can open and close. When the gates are open, the pain reaches your brain and you feel it. When the gates are closed, the pain is blocked from reaching the brain, so you feel it less or maybe even not at all.

We still don't know exactly how the nerve gates work, but

we do know we can influence them by interfering with the pain signals through spinal cord stimulation, also called neurostimulation. If your foot hurts and someone bites you on the hand, for instance, your foot won't hurt so much because now you've got another pain message coming in that blocks the one from your foot.

I don't recommend biting yourself as a treatment, so instead, we use an electronic device that's basically a small box about the size of your palm that contains a battery and a miniaturized computer. A little paddle about the size of a paper clip is attached to it by a wire. The device is surgically implanted just under the skin. The paddle is placed next to the spinal cord, usually somewhere at the level of the ribcage. The box goes just under the skin above your buttocks or in your abdomen near the belly button. The computer tells the battery to generate a mild electric pulse that's transmitted through the wire to the paddle. It works in much the same way as a pacemaker device for your heart, except it has an on-off switch that you control.

The mild electric stimulation interferes with the pain message and keeps it from getting to your brain. Is it blocking the signal or just changing your sensation and interpretation of the pain? We don't know—we just know that it helps some patients. Some get complete pain relief, but most get only partial relief. Just cutting your pain in half, however, is generally enough to make it much more tolerable. You need fewer painkillers and your function improves.

Spinal cord stimulation is a safe and effective technique that has been FDA approved since 1989. It's particularly effective for helping people with continuing pain from failed back surgery. I like to use a temporary external device first to make sure it's going to help before we go ahead and do the very simple procedure for implanting the device. I use a local anesthetic, put the lead into the right area, and apply electrical stimulation from the outside, without implanting the generator box. After a few days, we have a good idea of whether it's helping or not. If it doesn't, I can remove the lead painlessly in the office and just give you a little bandage over the insertion point.

MEDICATION MANAGEMENT

We back surgeons and pain doctors are often blamed for starting the opioid epidemic by overprescribing narcotic pain drugs. I would dispute that strenuously, but the issue of opioids is an important one. No responsible doctor wants to prescribe something with an addiction risk unless it's absolutely necessary. In some cases, it is. For a patient in very severe pain, I will sometimes prescribe a powerful opiate for very short-term use. Beyond that, the pain can and should be managed through less powerful drugs and nonsurgical methods, unless it is clearly a case where surgery is needed. In some cases, however, longer-term use of opiates is needed. If I am certain this is the only way to go for a particular patient, I will prescribe the drugs. I'll also refer the patient to a pain specialist for further treatment and ongoing management because they have the experience to help.

LONG-TERM USE OF PAIN DRUGS

I had an older lady with stenosis in her lower spine who was worried about becoming addicted to her pain drugs. She wanted to be off of them. I asked what she took for her pain and how she felt when she didn't take her medicine. She said if she didn't take it, she was always thinking about her medicine and in constant pain throughout the day. That's the sort of answer that suggests addiction, but when I asked her how much medication she took, she replied, "I take half a Percocet [acetaminophen with oxycodone] in the morning, and in about 15 minutes I feel really good. I might get a little sore in the afternoon and I'll either take an ibuprofen pill or maybe take another half Percocet. Does that mean I'm addicted?" "No," I told her. "You're far from being addicted because you use the same dose all the time and don't need more. You're just controlling your pain very sensibly." For patients like this one, long-term use of low-dose painkillers is safe and appropriate.

Many drugs that aren't addictive painkillers are very helpful for managing back pain. The standard over-the-counter nonsteroidal anti-inflammatory drugs (NSAIDs), such as ibuprofen (Advil, Motrin) and naprosyn (Aleve) can be very helpful. Surprisingly, acetaminophen (Tylenol), which isn't an anti-inflammatory, is still a very good pain-relieving medicine for most people. We can also cautiously use prescription-strength NSAIDs such as celecoxib (Celebrex).

A mild prescription muscle relaxant such as cyclobenzaprine (Flexeril) can help loosen muscle spasms and block pain impulses. It's meant for short-term use of no more than a few weeks. I often prescribe it to patients who are in too much pain to do physical therapy. The drug relaxes the muscles enough so that they can begin working with their therapist.

Sometimes a low dose of an antidepressant drug can help with pain. We can also try drugs designed to treat pain by calming down irritated nerves, such as gabapentin (Neurontin) and amitriptyline (Elavil). These drugs can cause drowsiness, dizziness, and other side effects, although these are usually minimal because we use only a low dose. They only work in about half of all patients, but I can't tell in advance if they'll work for you. We have to just try one and see if it reduces your pain.

Multimodal therapy, where we use drugs in combination, can be more helpful than just a big dose of one drug. Ibuprofen plus acetaminophen, for example, seems to work better in combination than either drug alone. For a lot of people, the combination works as well as an opioid drug, without the drawbacks.

PHYSICAL THERAPY

Of all the nonoperative techniques that can help relieve back pain, physical therapy is one of the best—and the most challenging for patients. PT isn't like an injection or a pill. You have to actively participate in PT for it to work.

Physical therapy focuses on teaching you how to do specific exercises to strengthen your muscles and specific ways of moving to help heal your back and prevent reinjury. A lot of the exercise work is to increase your range of motion and get your movement back in balance. Your physical therapist will also focus on teaching you how to stand and sit better, how to lift things to avoid hurting your back, and workplace and home ergonomics, or ways to move and work more safely and comfortably. I prescribe physical therapy for just about all my patients, whether or not they're going to have surgery. In fact, most health insurers won't pay for your back surgery unless you've done serious PT first. If you do need surgery, PT before helps get you into the best shape possible; afterward, it's a must to build up muscle strength and get your body balanced again.

Physical therapy can also help decrease acute inflammation and get you through the painful acute phase of a back injury. Your physical therapist will apply ice or heat to the painful area and then help you stretch through it to loosen up the muscles and improve your range of motion. If you have arthritis in your hand, for instance, your physical therapist may have you dip your hand in a hot wax bath to get deep heat to the joints. That loosens them up so that you can move on to do hand exercises.

When you go for your first PT session, the therapist will start by examining you. They want to see your range of motion and figure out where you're hurting. This is an important step because it helps them design an individualized treatment program. You don't want your therapist to say, "Oh, you've got back pain, here's an exercise, do that for 10 minutes, I'll be right back." Find someone else if that happens. The physical therapist needs to examine you, ideally agree with the diagnosis you've been sent to them for, and come up with a treatment plan. The plan should start by taking care of the acute issues through range of motion and stretching exercises and modalities such as heat, ice, and massage. Those treatments will get you through the initial phase and help reduce the inflammation and pain.

When you're feeling better, your therapist will move you on to the active phase. This is where you learn how to move again. The therapist will work on your proprioception, or your ability to know where your body is. Often, after an injury or if you've been moving or walking in a distorted way because your back hurts, your body is out of alignment. You need to relearn subconsciously where your body really is. Where you think your left leg is, the one that hurts from sciatica, may not be quite where it actually is. You need to reprogram your body to know where it is and how it's moving. If you've been walking funny for a while to accommodate your back pain, you need help to reverse that now that the pain is better. That will also help with the knee or hip trouble you might now be having from walking in a distorted way and putting extra pressure on those joints.

Going to PT is a lot like going to the gym. Your therapist will work with you on active balancing exercises, muscle strengthening, and core exercises. The facility has gym mats, exercise bikes, treadmills, weights, and lots of other equipment designed to help you build strength. Physical therapists love exercise bands, so they have big rolls of special colored rubber tapes they use to make them for you.

The goal of the first few sessions of PT is to help you feel better for a short period of time through stretching and the other modalities. After that, though, the goal is to build up your coordination for whole-body exercises—this is a much more active phase of the program. I want you to sweat during a PT session, and I want you to feel it in mildly sore muscles afterward. I want you to work hard at the PT center and at home when you do the exercises your therapist teaches you. Think of the therapists as instructors who are teaching you things you will do for the rest of your life, not just as massage therapists.

When I prescribe PT, I give the therapist some general

guidance about what to work on and how many sessions I think it will take. I might recommend core strengthening exercises and maybe dry needling for muscle spasms, but in general, I give the therapists some latitude about how to work with you. These people are very well trained to work with the diagnosis in the best way. I leave it to the therapist to work with the patient on the best exercises to deal with a lumbar strain, for example.

When the PT session is over and you've worked hard, you might be feeling it—a flare-up of pain isn't uncommon. That's when your physical therapist will probably put heat on the area and use the ultrasound machine and a gel to push the heat deeper into the muscle. That opens up the blood flow, which brings more oxygen to the area and carries away waste products. Heat is very soothing to aching muscles. Some people prefer to use ice. That's fine—your therapist can provide ice packs.

A prescription for PT is generally for six to eight weeks. For the first few weeks, you'll probably be going two to three times a week, but toward the end of the sessions, when you've learned how to do the exercises and have established a good pattern of doing them at home, you'll need to go just once a week. The therapist will want to see you to be sure you're using good form for the home exercises.

For patients recovering from surgery, I'll sometimes recommend water therapy. Because you're in a pool, the treatment is less painful—the water supports you and the buoyancy makes you feel the tug of gravity less. It helps patients who are concerned about falling in those first few weeks after surgery.

We know that most people will get better without surgery. Once we have the best diagnosis we can find and we've done things like injections to calm down the inflammation, we want to get you moving safely again in a way that doesn't make the pain worse and keeps you from reinjuring yourself. The best way to do that is with physical therapy. You work with a skilled professional in a safe, controlled environment to get back to your normal activities. For many of my patients, that means using muscles they haven't used in a long time. We need to build all their muscles and get them back in shape.

The beauty of physical therapy isn't just that it helps. Your physical therapist will guide you through the exercises, stretches, and retraining it takes to help you be responsible for your own health. They'll teach you what to do, but it's up to you to do it at home in between sessions. Once the sessions end, it's up to you to do those exercises faithfully to keep your back pain manageable.

Some orthopedic practices also own physical therapy practices and will refer you there because they know the staff are very capable. You don't have to go where the doctor suggests, however. Often, the practices I recommend in my area aren't convenient for my patients, who may come long distances to see me. I'd much rather you find a physical therapy center near you and go regularly. A good starting point is your local hospital, which may have a PT practice.

Occasionally, a patient won't show any significant improvement after four or five weeks of PT. At that point, I recommend a change of treatments, a different therapist, or even a change to a different therapy center. Some centers aren't as aggressive as others in making you work hard. A different PT may be better at picking the right exercises for you and motivating you to do your home exercises. A PT is like a personal trainer in many ways, and you need to have a good rapport.

In recent years, an exciting new nonoperative approach to back pain has come into use: regenerative medicine. Stem cells and other regenerative therapies have enormous potential—so enormous that I'll spend all of the next chapter discussing their use.

CHAPTER 6

Regenerative Therapies

Roller derby is a fun sport to watch and to play, but it's also a full-contact sport that carries a high risk of injury. Because I have a reputation for treating back injuries from sports, the local roller derby queens often come to me. I recently had a patient who had a serious contusion (bad bruise) and some torn ligaments right along the iliac crest on one side—that's the top part of your hip bone where your belt line is. Three months later, she was still having pain in the area. She'd tried everything—anti-inflammatory drugs, heat, rest, local injections of steroids—but nothing helped. I decided to try a regenerative therapy: injections of platelet-rich plasma to spur the healing process. They worked well. Within a couple of weeks, she was able to get back to her normal life and also to roller derby.

REGENERATING THE BODY

Regenerative medicine uses a range of techniques to regrow, repair, or replace damaged or diseased cells, organs, or tissues. This approach to treating injury and disease has been around for a long time. We've been successfully replacing hearts, kidneys, and other organs for decades. The first successful kidney transplant, for instance, was in 1954. More recently, we've started using stem cells and other techniques, such as platelet-rich plasma, to treat bone, cartilage, and connective tissue problems. We're now able to restore some degenerating tissues by using stem cells to induce bone and connective tissue growth. We've had great success with using stem cells to help with arthritic knees.

STEM CELLS

Stem cells are cells within your body that have the amazing ability to divide indefinitely and develop into many different types of cells. Stem cells are particularly important during early life when the body grows rapidly. Later in life, they act as the body's internal repair system. Each time a stem cell divides, it has the potential to become a specialized type of cell, such as a muscle cell or cartilage. In adults, stem cells regenerate some tissues that are lost through normal wear and tear or injury, such as muscle, brain, and bone marrow cells. These are tissues that don't regenerate themselves—your body relies on its supply of stem cells to turn into new cells.

What makes stem cells so valuable for regenerative medicine is that, under the right conditions, we can induce a stem cell to become a specific type of cell with the special functions that cell has. So, we can, under the right circumstances, make a stem cell become a muscle cell or a cartilage cell.

EPIGENETICS

Epigenetics is the study of how the environment around your genes affects their expression. For example, you might be genetically prone to getting lung cancer. But if you don't smoke and avoid second-hand smoke, the environment around your genes is free of the substances that trigger your lung cells to start reproducing uncontrollably. The genes that cause cancer aren't triggered to express themselves. In the larger picture, epigenetics is why we can potentially pass on certain characteristics to our offspring. We're passing on not just our genetic code, but the expression of the code. This is why maternal nutrition, for instance, plays a big role in how the offspring do in life. Good nutrition for the mother means the child's genetic code gets expressed well; poor nutrition can distort the expression in damaging ways that last a lifetime.

Part of the key of regenerative therapy includes acknowledging that we're not doomed to be what our genes say we are. The genetic code has a lot of redundancy, so if one gene isn't expressed well or even at all, others can provide a similar function. How we grow and what our potential is can be affected by what we eat, and also by the overall environment, how much stress we have, how much sunlight we get, what our communities are like, how much and what sort of exercise we get. Exercise doesn't just build muscles, it teaches the cells in those muscles to express their genes in a particular way.

The impact of epigenetics affects your entire body and even your lifespan. Residents of some cities in Italy have fewer heart attacks than residents of other cities. The reason is probably the epigenetic effect of stress on the body. In the cities where people feel a stronger sense of community and have more social bonds, fewer people have heart attacks. The theory is that less stress from a more socially supportive environment leads to fewer stress hormones and less inflammation, which means less hardening of the arteries and fewer heart attacks.

By optimizing our health environment, we can change the ways our genes are expressed. When someone does physical therapy, changes their diet, and changes their sleep schedule, it helps them heal from back pain. But at a more fundamental level, those changes affect the way their genes are expressed. In a way, it's almost like giving them brand-new genes.

If we look at regenerative medicine as including the epigenetic effect of the environment, you want to optimize your personal health environment. There are a number of ways to do this.

OPTIMIZE YOUR DIET

Top of the list is optimizing your diet to reduce inflammation, as I explained back in chapter 2. A good example of how diet can affect the genes is treating some forms of epilepsy with a ketogenic diet—a diet that is relatively high in fat and protein and very low in carbohydrates. The diet forces the body to burn ketones, not glucose, as its primary fuel. In fact, a ketogenic diet was the primary therapy for epilepsy until anticonvulsant drugs were developed in the 1920s. When doctors started relying on these drugs, which can have some very unpleasant side effects, they forgot about the ketogenic diet. The diet modifies the expression of the genes that are responsible for epilepsy.

GET MICRONUTRIENTS

The next step in optimizing your diet is to get plenty of micronutrients by eating a wide variety of fresh foods, including lots of colorful fruits and vegetables. You need to maintain a good balance of omega-3 and omega-6 fatty acids and get plenty of vitamin D from supplements or sunlight.

You also need plenty of vitamin C. Very few people these

days get scurvy, the deficiency disease causes by lack of vitamin C. Just about everyone gets the bare minimum amount of about 50 mg a day needed to prevent that, but a surprising number of people don't get the RDA of 95 mg a day. They don't eat enough fresh fruit and vegetables to get an adequate dietary intake. After all, there isn't much vitamin C in a burger and fries, even if you wash it down with an orange soda. Other micronutrients, such as magnesium and zinc, need to be optimized through supplements because modern farming methods have reduced the mineral content of the soil.

HYPERBARIC OXYGEN THERAPY

Hyperbaric oxygen therapy is a way to use pressure to force more oxygen into your cells. Most people think of hyperbaric treatment as way to treat the bends, which happens to divers who ascend from deep water too quickly. To treat the bends, you go into a hyperbaric chamber, a sealed compartment that can be pressurized by pumping in air and added oxygen.

We can also use hyperbaric oxygen therapy for treating conditions that would be helped by getting more oxygen to the tissues. Post-op wounds heal faster if we do hyperbaric therapy. Wounds that won't heal can also be helped by this therapy. It's possible that it also helps any problem that involves tissues that don't normally get a lot of oxygen, such as the discs in your spinal column, and can help heal nerve injuries.

BIOLOGICAL ADJUNCTS

Optimizing health may include replacing or supplementing some hormones. We do this all the time for some conditions, such as severe osteoporosis. That can be treated with a drug called teriparatide (Forteo), which is parathyroid hormone (your parathyroid glands produce a hormone that controls the level of calcium in your body). Forteo stimulates your body to build new bone and increase bone density.

Many women use bioidentical hormone replacement therapy during and after menopause. We know that women who are on these hormones decrease their rate of gastrointestinal cancer by 50 percent. They decrease their risk of age-related macular degeneration (vision loss) significantly. They can decrease their risk of vascular disease, including Alzheimer's, if they maintain good levels of estrogen and progesterone.

A lot of men now use testosterone replacement therapy, although this must be used cautiously. Recent studies refute the idea of testosterone supplementation increasing heart attacks, but it is one reason you should consult with an up-to-date doctor to see what the current understanding of different treatments is.

The thyroid gland also secretes a hormone which is essential for healing and growth. Those who have low thyroid hormones often have weight gain, dry skin, hair loss, constipation, fatigue, muscle weakness, and a feeling of being cold. Many women and some men have low thyroid function, and supplemental hormones are often prescribed to compensate.

Numerous studies suggest that taking human growth hormone (HGH) if your levels are low is a good idea. Most people don't need a pharmacologic dose (an amount significantly higher than what your body would make), just a dose just large enough to bring your level back to the normal range. Exactly what the normal range is can be controversial, but the idea is that if you raise your HGH level, you'll have better health and repair. Importantly, you'll maintain your current muscle mass and bone strength against the slow loss that inevitably comes with age.

You can naturally stimulate your production of these hormones through a low-carb diet, weight training, aerobic exercise, adequate sleep, and other positive lifestyle changes. Supplements might not be needed, but it is important to achieve optimal hormone levels for ideal healing and overall health and wellness.

PROLOTHERAPY

Let's say you break your leg. When that happens, typically you'll have some bleeding near the fracture and the bone will move a little bit. A pocket of bleeding will form around the broken place and form a clot. The area is now full of platelets, the tiny particles in your blood that are part of the clotting process. The platelets send out chemical signals that, among other things, tell your body to start laying down demineralized bone cells that stick to the existing bone. Eventually, those cells calcify and become healed bone. That would be a normal response for bone healing.

Similarly, if you sprain your ankle and injure a tendon (the tough tissue that attaches muscle to bone) or a ligament (the tough tissue that attaches bone to bone in a joint), there's typically some bleeding, which is why the area is bruised. Again, a clot forms and the platelets send chemical signals that tell your body to build up collagen in the injured area to heal it.

Sometimes, maybe because of poor blood supply or inactivity or poor nutrition, that healing process is very slow. It might end too soon or not really happen at all. One way to try to get the healing process moving is to start it all over again by simulating an injury and irritating the area. Prolotherapy, as this is called, uses needles inserted into the area where the ligament or tendon hasn't healed. A harmless fluid, usually dextrose (sugar water), is then injected around the joint. Your body responds by saying, "Wow, that's irritating. Let's get rid of that." The irritation jump-starts the stalled natural healing process. Prolotherapy is a shorthand way of saying proliferation therapy; it's also called regenerative injection therapy.

Sometimes, when a damaged ligament stays inflamed and is slow to heal, we use a similar technique called barbotage. This procedure makes you into a sort of pincushion by giving you a lot of little injections of lidocaine or some steroid into the area to calm the inflammation. We back the needle in and out, in and out, around the area to cause just a little bit of bleeding. That brings in platelets to get the healing moving again.

Back pain has a lot of causes beyond disc herniation. When the pain is coming from the spinous process (the bumps you feel in your back when you touch your spine), it may be due to injury to the tendons and muscles that attach to them. Sometimes prolotherapy or barbotage can get the healing process to move faster. The sacroiliac joint is held together with a lot of ligaments. When the joint is very inflamed, we can try prolotherapy or barbotage to calm it down. The area doesn't have much blood supply, so stimulating it to bring platelets to the area can help.

The idea behind prolotherapy is that injections into the painful area will help promote healing of a ligament or tendon. The goal is to strengthen weakened connective tissue and improve musculoskeletal pain. While prolotherapy won't help nerve issues such as pain from the pressure of a herniated disc, it can be particularly helpful for sacroiliac (SI) joint dysfunction. This painful condition is usually caused by abnormal movement—either too much or too little—within the joint. The ligaments in the joint are often the cause of the problem. Prolotherapy can help heal the ligaments and muscles and decrease excessive movement in the SI joint.

To do prolotherapy, we inject a small amount of a dextrose solution, which is sugar water, mixed with a local anesthetic into the ligaments, using image guidance to make sure we place it properly. The dextrose isn't a drug; it's just a safe way to irritate the ligament. Most patients need around four to six treatments to feel better, but some people need as many as ten treatments. The injections do hurt as they go in, and there's some pain in the area for a few hours after, but most patients find the discomfort very tolerable.

COLD AND HEAT THERAPY

Cold immersion is becoming popular among professional athletes as a way to recover more quickly from strenuous workouts and injuries. It's done by sitting in very cold water for a short period after training hard. By some reports, this reduces inflammation so much that recovery time improves from five or six days to just one.

Taking a cold shower every day can help decrease total body inflammation, help build more mitochondria, and can help decrease excess fat and body weight.

The heat from saunas has been shown to help reduce inflammation and improve cardiovascular function. Saunas may even increase longevity in people who use them frequently. Everyone should use this—I certainly do.

BONE GRAFTING

Bone grafting is another aspect of using your own cells to heal the body. We use bone grafts to stimulate bones that are slow to heal or aren't healing at all. Bone from one part of the body is moved to the damaged area, often to make the bones there fuse together. The techniques we use for bone grafts today are very different from in the past. Patients could have pain from the donor site for as long as a year afterward. Today, we use minimally invasive techniques that cause less pain. We take the bone for the graft from the iliac crest in the hip area, because when we remove a small piece there, we know it will grow back well and won't interfere with your life while it does. The bone graft from the iliac crest has good marrow in it, which means lots of cells to stimulate the healing. Today, we have additional techniques for fusing bones and cells that work better and don't cause a lot of pain at the donor site. Instead, I use a big needle to suck some marrow out of the iliac crest and mix those cells in with the artificial bone we now use. The live cells increase the healing speed.

PLATELET-RICH PLASMA

Sometimes I'll give a patient an injection of steroids and local anesthetic into a painful area. If the injection helps, I know I've found the source of the pain. But if the pain comes back quickly, it's often a sign that the steroid helped a bit, but the inflammation in the area is more than the amount I inject can help. That's an indication that platelet-rich plasma (PRP) could help. By injecting some of the patient's own platelets directly into the painful area, we can accelerate the healing process. The platelets send out chemical signals to the body, telling it to produce more natural anti-inflammatory substances in the area.

To get the platelets, I draw some blood from your arm. The procedure only needs about 15 to 50 ml, or less than two ounces. The blood is put into a centrifuge and spun around until it separates out into different layers. The layer with the platelets in it is what we want. It's very concentrated, which is why it's called platelet-rich plasma. The PRP is then injected, very precisely, often using X-ray or ultrasound guidance into the damaged portion of the tendon or ligament. Ordinarily, not that many platelets get to these points, so by adding a concentrated number of them, healing is stimulated in a way your body can't. The platelets think they're at that part of the body because they need to heal an injury—they get to work producing those natural healing substances.

Because we use your own blood for this technique and don't process the platelets in any way, PRP is a very safe technique when done by an experienced doctor. I have to be honest here and say that getting the injection does hurt a bit, but it's nothing horrible. Patients tell me that they can feel their existing pain when the needle goes in. That's good because it tells me I've got the right spot. PRP isn't a miracle cure. I do it only if nothing else has helped so far—it's not a first-line treatment, although some elite athletes do use it that way. PRP can take several weeks to work and you may need more than one treatment. Sometimes it doesn't work at all and sometimes the relief isn't permanent. But even if you get pain relief for just a year or so, in the meantime, you've got decreased pain and improved function. That's worthwhile by itself, but it could also mean that you can do physical therapy more effectively.

PRP is also being used to help stimulate the subcutaneous tissue to build more collagen and other soft tissue. In the face, this thickens the area under the skin and makes it firmer. When these injections are done for cosmetic reasons around the face, fewer wrinkles and a more youthful look can be the result. More and more applications of PRP are being discovered all the time. This is another reason to ask an experienced doctor more about these procedures.

PLATELET-POOR PLASMA

If, instead of using the concentrated platelets from a patient's blood, and we took them out, we're left with platelet-poor plasma. This liquid has concentrated amounts of healing elements and hormones that can improve healing. When we spray this on the edges of surgical incisions when we're sewing them back together, the wound heals a little faster with less scarring. Platelet-poor plasma can also be injected into the epidural space around a vertebra. That's being researched now as a way to possibly decrease pain or increase healing.

STEM CELL THERAPY

Stem cells are pluripotent, meaning they can turn into any type of more specialized cells. They're found throughout the body, including in the bone marrow. They're also found in the tiny blood vessels that run through body fat. Wherever they are, stem cells seem to just sit there, waiting until something in the body gets injured and they're needed to repair it.

Stem cell therapy is based on the idea that injecting stem cells into an injured area stimulates them to turn into the right sort of cells to heal the injury by replacing the damaged cells. If we inject stem cells into the knee joint of someone with osteoarthritis, for example, they may grow into cartilage cells. We're finding that injecting stem cells into ligaments, tendons, muscles, or even the discs seems to help them regenerate.

Stem cell therapy can be extremely helpful in the right situations, but it's still considered experimental by most health insurance plans. In the U.S., the FDA says we can do stem cell therapy only if we use your own stem cells, drawn from your body, minimally processed, and injected back into you. To do this, we take the stem cells found in the bone marrow of the iliac crest of your hip bone. There's nothing special about the iliac crest stem cells, it's just that this is an easily accessible part of your body for harvesting them. We concentrate the marrow to get the stem cells out and then inject them into wherever we want the healing to go. The hope is that the stem cells will recognize that they're needed and will start turning into whatever type of cells are required.

As with PRP, this treatment doesn't always work. It gives your body one last chance to heal on its own. We do it when we've tried other techniques that haven't worked well. It's the last option to try before surgery. A fair number of my patients who have tried this have achieved significant improvement in their back pain, to the point where six months afterward, they have healed enough to decide against surgery. I've seen numbers saying that 90 percent of patients say they feel better, but I'm skeptical. In my experience, about 70 to 80 percent of patients say they're better. That's still pretty darn good.

The best candidate for stem cell therapy is someone who's relatively young (under 60) and has a ligament problem. Older adults have fewer stem cells in general and their discs are usually so worn out that stem cells won't help. Yet these days, people are taking care of themselves, and their bodies may be "staying younger" longer. So people who are older can be considered for this kind of stem cell treatment.

When I inject you with stem cells, you feel the pressure, which can be uncomfortable at the time. The procedure can make you hurt more for the first few weeks because we've put a bunch of cells into a confined space. That creates pressure and some pain. The stem cells take about six months to work. If you're not feeling noticeably better by then, you probably won't. Unfortunately, the procedure hasn't worked for you and you're now back to thinking about surgery. The good news is that stem cell treatment doesn't burn any bridges. It doesn't affect your ability to have successful surgery because the treatment hasn't done any further damage.

If you've tried to heal your back using everything I've discussed in this book so far, and nothing has helped for long, surgery may be your next step.

CHAPTER 7

Precision Laser Surgeries

You've worked closely with your doctor, done your physical therapy faithfully, and tried other nonsurgical approaches to your back pain. It's still there—in fact, the pain is getting worse. Now what?

It may be time to visit a spine surgeon and explore the surgical options. As a spine surgeon, I know surgery can help, sometimes dramatically, but it's not a miracle cure. I recommend seeing a very experienced surgeon, asking a lot of questions, and thinking carefully about your expectations and your commitment to physical therapy during your recovery before you decide on surgery for back pain.

To help you understand the options your surgeon offers, in this chapter I'll explain the various precision techniques we can use to perform minimally invasive surgery and get you back on your feet fast.

ADVANTAGES OF MINIMALLY INVASIVE SURGERY

Minimally invasive surgery (MIS) has many advantages for patients. It's fast—it's frequently done on an outpatient basis. You arrive at the hospital or surgery center first thing in the morning and you usually go home in the afternoon. Today's anesthesia techniques mean you wake up and get back to normal function fast. An overnight stay in the hospital is rarely needed. In general, MIS lets you bleed less, go home faster, and heal quicker.

With MIS, there's no need for big incisions and stitches, bulky bandages, bed rest, body casts, or heavy-duty pain meds. We can reach the area of the spine that needs work in ways that avoid touching other nerves and that minimize cutting through muscle. MIS is often called Band-Aid surgery because the incisions are so small. Because the anesthesia and surgery are less stressful to your body, you recover and heal better and faster.

In the past, spine surgery used to be very bloody. Bone and muscle would bleed to the point where you could lose a liter or two of blood and need a transfusion. A major advantage of minimally invasive surgery is that it bleeds a lot less. The vast majority of patients don't need blood transfusions. We use a machine called a cell saver to collect the blood lost during surgery, clean it up, and transfuse it back into you if needed—but it rarely is.

One of the great things about minimally invasive surgery is sometimes I don't do everything the imaging suggests. I'll ask you about your symptoms and focus on them for your surgery, even if something on the imaging looks suspicious. We can do that because with MIS, we're not burning any bridges by causing scar tissue or destabilization that would make a second surgery a real problem. If something else becomes an issue later on, we can just do another surgery to address that. Sometimes we choose to do less to get good results and avoid a larger surgery. That's something you and your surgeon need to work out.

The surgery may be outpatient, but that doesn't mean you're ready to go dancing the same day. Your pain right after the procedure won't be severe, however, and it will be very manageable without heavy-duty opioids over the next few days. After that, the pain will probably be minimal and will almost certainly be gone within two weeks. The incision for minimally invasive surgery, by definition, is small and cuts through very few muscles. That helps keep the pain down, reduces scarring, and leads to a faster recovery. You're able to start your physical therapy program soon after the surgery.

Let me repeat that: you'll be able to start your physical

therapy program soon after the surgery. Doing your PT is crucial to your recovery. I ask my patients to make a real commitment to it before I agree to operate.

IS SURGERY RIGHT FOR YOU?

When I evaluate a patient for possible surgery, I'm looking at some fundamental issues. I want to be sure that the surgery will improve or resolve them, take away most or even all your pain, and leave you with good range of motion. In surgery, I want to:

- Decompress any spinal nerves that are being pinched or pressured by a bulging or collapsed disc, arthritis, or bone spurs.
- Stabilize your spine.
- Realign and balance your spine if needed.
- Preserve your ability to move comfortably and be active.
- Decrease your pain.

The surgery for decompressing and stabilizing your spine usually involves one or more of these procedures:

- Laminotomy or laminectomy. Removing a part or all of the bony arch (lamina) of the damaged area of the spinal canal as a way to increase the size of the canal and relieve pressure on the nerves—that's why this surgery is also called a disc decompression. We use a small incision to remove a little bit of the lamina, the thin layer of bone that forms a roof over the spinal cord. We basically make a little window in the lamina so we can see the damaged disc. If just a section of the lamina is removed, it's a laminotomy. If I have to take out the entire lamina, it's a laminectomy.

- Discectomy. Removing some or all of the damaged disc to relieve the pressure on the affected nerves. The nerve is moved to one side and then the herniated part of the disc is removed.
- Foraminotomy or foraminectomy. Expanding the opening where the nerve roots leave the spinal canal (the foramen) by removing a small amount of bone and tissue. If I have to remove a lot of bone and tissue to enlarge the opening, it's called a foraminectomy.
- Osteophyte removal. In this procedure, bone spurs (osteophytes) that are pressing on a nerve are removed.
- Fusion. To stabilize the spine at the painful place and keep it from moving, we link two or sometimes more vertebrae together, using a bone graft or bone cage and screws, rods, and other hardware to hold them in place. The vertebrae fuse together, forming one solid bone instead of a mobile joint.

BONE CAGES

Anterior interbody cages, called bone cages for short, are porous cylinders or rectangles made of titanium or plastic. A bone cage is placed in the disc space to hold the vertebrae apart after the damaged disc has been removed. The cage is packed with bone graft to stimulate bone growth. The bone grows in through the holes in the cage from the vertebral bodies above and below it, fusing the vertebrae together. The cage becomes part of your spine.

FUSION SURGERY

Fusion surgery is primarily used to treat problems with the discs, including:

- Degenerative disc disease
- Disc herniation
- Radiculopathy
- Spinal stenosis
- Foraminal stenosis
- Spinal segmental instability
- Scoliosis and spinal curvature deformity

STAGED SURGERY

Sometimes I recommend staged surgery, where I follow one surgery with another at a later date. I might do a decompression of a nerve to relieve leg pain because that's the immediate problem, let the patient fully recover, and save the bigger surgery to fix the curve in the spine for when it's needed more. Patients sometimes say, "As long as you're under the hood, doc, can't you fix everything?" I explain that minimally invasive surgery is like my airplane engine. To check the oil, I open a little window in the cowling to see the gauge. But to check the spark plugs, I have to take the whole cowling off. That's like back surgery. I can see into the little window of your spine for the decompression procedure, but to do others at the same time involves a lot more cutting. I have to make a surgical plan and focus on that. The good thing about MIS is that it leaves very little scarring and you recover fast. If I need to do another procedure later, it's not a problem the way it would be with big, open surgery. Sometimes smaller surgeries with fast recovery times in between are better than one big surgery.

SURGICAL TECHNIQUES

Before the surgery, I use computer reconstruction and animation to plan out what I'm going to do. The tools I use during a minimally invasive surgery are amazing. I use microscopes, loupes, and magnifying lenses to see the area in remarkable detail and cut only where I need to, using minimal incisions. I use tiny instruments inserted through retractors, so the incision is very small, often under an inch long.

Additional tools I can use include robots, computer imaging, laser guidance, and other techniques that help with some surgeries. Once I've decided, based on my examination, all the precision imaging, and your symptoms that spine surgery is the right thing for you, I can make a recommendation about the best way to proceed. The final decision on what to do is made jointly by the patient with me. We consider your needs and goals when deciding what procedure is best for you.

PRECISION LASER SURGERY

I use lasers in minimally invasive surgery to provide a form of very precise heat that's especially useful for shrinking collagen in discs. Laser surgery has become a synonym for minimally invasive surgery not because we use lasers a lot, but because laser is a shorthand way of saying high-tech. Minimally invasive surgery uses extremely cool high-tech tools. One way I use lasers in every surgery is in the X-ray fluoroscopy that's so important for reaching exactly the right area. To cut down on the radiation, I expose the patient and the operating room staff to, I use lasers to point to exactly the spot I want to X-ray. I also use lasers for aligning things like screws and rods during surgery. These lasers are basically high-tech versions of the little laser gadgets you can buy to help you hang pictures on a wall.

ROBOTIC SURGERY

I will often use robotic-assisted surgery. Additionally, 2-D and 3-D computer-generated images can be reconstructed and used with Virtual Reality (VR) or Augmented Reality (AR) to perform surgery with very small incisions. With these tools, I can either see a representation of the spinal anatomy on a screen (VR), or see "through" the patient, through the skin, to see the spine in Augmented Reality (AR) and use this information directly during surgery. Robots, 3-D images generated by computer, and images augmented by computer are tools which are now available for surgeries—and they continue to improve.

We are quite a ways from doing surgeries remotely or from having robots doing the entire surgery. Yet we are making progress. The assistance robots and virtual reality give me in surgery can help surgery become even safer and less invasive.

ENDOSCOPIC SURGERY AND BESS

Somewhere in the transition between percutaneous procedures like Rhizotomies, BVN ablation, injections, and other types of outpatient procedures—and between more open surgical procedures (even when they are done in a minimally invasive fashion), are the endoscopic guided procedures.

Years ago, knee surgeries and shoulder surgeries in orthopedics, and gallbladder and appendix surgeries were done with larger open procedures. Today, many of these procedures are performed with small incisions, a microscopic camera, and instruments which are placed via small puncture incisions in order to do the surgery. Looking into joints (arthroscopic surgery) or into the abdomen (endoscopic surgery) with these scopes, and then doing the work, has become pretty common using techniques that have been developed over the past few decades.

Technology has advanced now where, for some diseases of the spine, a scope can be used with other tools through a small incision. These smaller incisions can be used to work in some very focused areas of the spine.

We can place a scope near or into the foramen, where the nerve comes out, and then make the space bigger by removing a disc fragment that shouldn't be there. Sometimes we can even shave some of the bone arthritis away to make more room for the nerve. A narrow tube with a couple of working channels can be placed at the foramen, using one channel to see with a camera, and through the other, the instruments can be placed to do the work required.

Or, we can use two arthroscopes (this is BESS, or bilateral endoscopic surgery) and create a small space to then do the work. In this case, two incisions are made, and the scope is used to see from a different angle than the working instrument. This affords some more visualization than a single portal. However, it can only be used in some of the larger spaces of the spine that have enough room for the instruments.

Endoscopic surgery of the spine is currently still in its infancy, yet is gaining more and more momentum. The equipment and techniques continue to advance and improve. While there were few indications for this procedure at one time, and as the instrumentation and the surgical skills advance, even more indications will follow.

FUSION TECHNIQUES

A number of techniques can be used to perform a lumbar spinal fusion. In most cases, I do a limited fusion, where I deal with one damaged or degenerated disc by fusing just two vertebrae together. After a limited fusion, you still usually have good range of motion and flexibility in the lower back, and your pain, numbness, tingling, and other symptoms are usually much better or gone. I do two-level or even three-level fusions when necessary, but only if this gives you a strong chance of improvement of the pain you came in with. I want to do the least amount of surgery that will help you. The relief from symptoms from multilevel fusion isn't that great, you lose a lot of mobility, and the extra stress on the other joints only leads to additional problems down the road.

INTERBODY FUSION

Interbody fusion means placing fusion implants (bone cages), made of titanium or plastic (or both), and bone graft into the area between two vertebrae to achieve fusion. I usually add bone healing protein to the area to encourage healing. One goal of the implant is to separate the vertebrae and hold them apart like the intervertebral disc used to do before it wore out. This enlarges the opening around the nerve roots and relieves pressure on them. Another goal is to realign the vertebrae to reproduce the normal curve of the spine.

Traditionally, the vertebrae were fused together with a bone graft, usually taken from the hip. Removing a wedge of bone from the hip was painful, however, and was a cause of surgical complications. The incision in the back needed to insert the graft was large. And most importantly, bone grafts often just didn't take. The nonunion rate (failure to fuse) was high.

Today, fusion is much less painful and much more likely to succeed. We use anterior interbody cages instead of bone wedge grafts from the hip. The cage is basically a threaded cylinder or a rectangle made of titanium or a type of plastic called PEEK. The cage is placed in the disc space between the vertebrae. The cage is porous and allows bone to grow through it and fuse the two vertebrae together. The process is helped along by putting screws connected by rods into the pedicles (the two stem-like structures that project from the back of the vertebra) to stabilize the joint and hold it in place. The beauty of the bone cage is that it's small. We can insert it using minimally invasive approaches. Once it's in place, the bone cage is held there by compression, which helps the bone fuse faster and better.

To further speed up healing and stimulate the bones to fuse, I often use a bone graft taken from the area being operated on (local bone). The bone is crushed into small chips and placed around the fusion site. Cells and proteins, along with the bone graft, stimulate the nearby bones to heal. If necessary, a larger chunk of bone is used to fill in the space where the removed disc used to be. I usually use your own bone (autograft), but when we need more bone than your own body can supply easily, I use donated bone from a cadaver (allograft).

In some cases, I also add bone morphogenic protein (BMP) to the area. BMP is the protein your body naturally makes to stimulate bone formation—it's what triggers stem cells to become bone cells. Recombinant human bone morphogenetic protein (rhBMP) is the genetically engineered equivalent. It's been approved by the FDA since 2002.

When I do a fusion surgery, I put some BMP on a sponge at the fusion site to help stimulate fusion between the vertebrae. BMP has basically eliminated the need for harvesting bone grafts from the hip. By using BMP, we've raised the fusion success rate to greater than 95 percent.

A common misperception about fusion surgery is that it makes your spine stiff and inflexible. Patients worry that they won't be able to bend over to tie their shoes or rotate their heads to look to the side. To some extent, that's true. After a fusion, you will be a bit stiffer. But you were already limited in your movement before the surgery, so if you end up with a little less motion, you're still much better off. Functionally, you might have more motion despite some stiffness in part of your spine. Before the surgery, you were in pain and your activity was very limited. After the surgery, you're feeling a lot better and your activity is limited a little bit, if at all. You haven't really sacrificed much, and you're back among the living in terms of being active again. If you've been having pain for a long time, it's possible that you've become very deconditioned and immobile from lack of activity. Your strength might be asymmetric and your range of motion might be disrupted. Surgery won't fix that—but it will make you mobile enough to do the physical therapy that will.

When your spine and the rest of your body are back to moving normally and you're back to having an active life, you'll feel so much better that you won't miss the couple of degrees of motion that are now gone. In fact, you might not notice the lost motion at all. I have patients who have had multiple fusions for scoliosis correction and can still bend over and put their palms on the ground because much of our range of motion is in our hips, not our lower back.

GOLFING BETTER

A lot of my patients are golfers. They come to me because their backs hurt too much to play, but many resist the idea of surgery because they fear they won't be able to get back in the game. I tell them they will probably play better after the surgery because they won't be in pain and they won't worry about hurting themselves every time they swing a club. Many of my golfing patients tell me that what they lose in power from the surgery, they gain in control. In fact, some become scratch golfers after the surgery.

LUMBAR SURGERIES

The lumbar region is the lower back, the part where the spine curves in toward the abdominal area. The lumbar spine has five vertebrae, designated L1 to L5. This part of the spine bears the most weight and is also the most prone to disc degeneration and other problems. Two basic approaches are used for minimally invasive lumbar surgery: anterior (from the front) and posterior (from the back).

ANTERIOR LUMBAR INTERBODY FUSION (ALIF)

When you think of spine surgery, you automatically think that it's done by cutting into your back. Historically, that was the case. We would do a posterior (from behind) lateral fusion, where we moved the back muscles to the side. We would then do a laminotomy or laminectomy to take the pressure off of the nerves. If fusion was needed, we would place the bone graft along either side of the spine where the facet joints are and hope it would take. Often, it didn't.

The posterior approach was needed because we had to have a big incision for the bone grafts on either side of the spine. Today, with bone cages and minimally invasive surgery, we can now approach the spine in other ways that involve fewer back muscles or don't involve them at all. (But as I'll explain later in this chapter, sometimes the traditional posterior approach is still necessary.)

Sometimes, the best way to do a back surgery is from the front (anterior). One way is the anterior lumbar interbody fusion (ALIF) to insert a bone cage. I like it because it lets me avoid the nerves from behind and get into the disc space between the vertebrae from the front part of the spine.

For this surgery, you need general anesthesia. You lie face up on a special surgical bed. The procedure is done through a 3-inch incision in your abdomen at the midline (the rectus muscle) just below your belly button. I use the incision to separate the fascia (the thin sheath of connective tissue that encloses a muscle) from the muscle. Using fluoroscopy or endoscopic imaging or computerized virtual reality, I then sneak around the rectus muscle, move the peritoneum (the sac that holds the intestines) to the side, and follow the inside walls of the abdominal cavity to get to the spine. I slide the big blood vessels to the side. Now I have a clear window to see the spine, using my magnifying lenses. I use tiny, surgical tools to remove the damaged disc, then I get the bony surfaces ready for the fusion. I spread them apart a bit to make room for the bone graft. This realigns the bones to the proper curvature and enlarges the openings to take the pressure off any pinched nerves.

The implant, filled with bone graft material, is placed in the now empty disc space between the two vertebrae. The bone graft inside the disc space will go on to fuse, healing the two bones together and forming a boney bridge to hold them in place. Once the fusion has healed, the two vertebrae will move as one unit. Sometimes I need to put a plate in from the front to hold the vertebrae in place. Sometimes I need to put screws and rods in from the back to do the same thing. I do this using either fluoroscopy or virtual imaging on a computer. The computer is very similar to using the Xbox Kinect®, where my gestures move the image around. I can even program a robot using virtual imaging to help put the screws in.

Some fusion patients have osteoporosis, which means

that they need some additional stabilization of the spine to make sure the vertebrae fuse together. In that case, the ALIF procedure is followed the next day by another procedure called posterior instrumentated fusion. In this procedure, some additional hardware to stabilize the spine is installed on the back of your spine.

A possible rare complication of ALIF surgery in men is retrograde ejaculation. This happens when the small nerves that control the valve that causes semen to be ejaculated outward are injured during the operation. The nerves temporarily keep the valve from working and make semen instead flow back into the bladder. Retrograde ejaculation doesn't affect your ability to have an erection or an orgasm, and it often goes away over time as the nerves heal. In rare cases, it stays and may cause male infertility.

The key reason the ALIF is so well tolerated is because we don't cut through any muscles. The incision in the abdomen goes through the skin and subcutaneous fat, but I don't cut any of the abdominal muscles. This means much less pain and a very quick recovery time.

XLIF AND DLIF

Sometimes we need to perform fusion surgery from a different approach. Another way to do an anterior surgery is to come from the side. The XLIF approach (extreme lateral interbody fusion) and the DLIF approach (direct lateral interbody fusion) are basically two names for the same surgical technique. For this surgery, you need general anesthesia. Because the incision is made into your side, not your abdomen, these approaches are a little less invasive. I don't have to avoid the great blood vessels, because they are already out of the way with this surgical approach. To reach the spine, I have to separate the three layers of muscles in your side. I do this by cutting through the fascia and then gently splitting the muscles with my finger, not cutting them with a scalpel. This spares the muscle strength and protects the nerves, so when I sew the fascia back, the muscles will be as strong as before. They won't hurt very much after the surgery.

The side approach doesn't work for everyone. It depends on your anatomy, the part of the spine I need to reach, how much spinal instability you have, and whether you've ever had any other surgery or radiation treatment in the abdominal area. I can't do this approach if I need to get to the lowest level of the spine (the sacrum), because your pelvic bone is in the way.

As with ALIF surgery, some patients may also need a posterior instrumentation and fusion.

OLIF

Another way to do an anterior surgery is to come from the

side using the OLIF approach (oblique lumbar interbody fusion). The OLIF in effect splits the difference between the ALIF and XLIF approaches and reaches the spine from a slightly different angle, usually about halfway between the midline and the side. Sometimes the oblique approach is the best way to get to the lowest lumbar discs because it lets me get around the iliac crest. In just about every other respect, the OLIF procedure is identical to the ALIF procedure. The only real difference is that you lie on your side, not your back, on the operating table. Also, coming in from an oblique approach allows me to work just anterior to the psoas muscle (ATP), which can be an advantage in people with large psoas muscles on either side of the spine—a muscle I often need to work through when using the DLIF/XLIF approach.

POSTERIOR LUMBAR SURGERY: TLIF AND PLIF

For some patients, reaching the spine from the back to fuse the vertebrae is still the best approach. TLIF (transforaminal lumbar interbody fusion) and PLIF (posterior lumbar interbody fusion) are both done from the back. This is a different approach from the ALIF etc.

The TLIF is done with either a traditional open incision or as a minimally invasive procedure (MIS)—the decision is based on what needs to be done. For this surgery, you will need general anesthesia. The procedure is a little different from an ALIF or a TLIF. Once I've reached the area where I want to be in the spine, I do a laminectomy—I remove the lamina so I can see the nerve roots. I may also cut away the facet joints to give the nerve roots more room. Then I move the nerve roots to one side so I can reach the disc space.

The damaged disc is removed, the bones are spread apart, the openings are enlarged, and the implant with bone graft is placed into the empty disc space to make the bones fuse together. Pedicle screws and rods are inserted to help with fixation and stability and help realign the spine to its normal curvature.

The transforaminal part of this procedure comes from the way I reach the foramen, or the opening around the nerves exiting the vertebrae. I reach underneath the nerves to enlarge the opening.

The advantage of the TLIF is that a larger surface area is available for the bone graft, which improves the likelihood of a successful fusion. The drawback is that the incision may need to be larger and I have to cut through the big muscles of the back.

The PLIF is basically the same as the TLIF, but a PLIF has a bilateral approach to the spine instead of from one side only.

A drawback to the TLIF and PLIF approaches is that these

surgeries can be a bit bloodier, but with minimally invasive techniques, the bleeding is reduced. I need to remove more bone and move through more muscle, so there's more bleeding. I can reduce the amount of damage to the muscles by gently splitting the muscles with my finger instead of cutting them with a scalpel. Sometimes the muscles have to be moved more to get to the spine, so you take a little longer to heal. MIS techniques limit the damage to the muscles.

The TLIF and PLIF approaches are most often used when, for some reason, I can't use the front or side approaches. If the patient has a big belly, for example, or has had previous surgery or radiation to the abdomen that has left a lot of scar tissue, I need to come in from the back instead. I also use the PLIF/TLIF approach if the nerves in the area need a lot of decompression.

For patients who have more complex needs, we can sometimes accomplish their goals in two steps. I do an anterior surgery first, wait for them to heal, and then do a later posterior surgery. Two smaller surgeries a few months apart can be better choice than one big surgery.

To decompress the nerves leaving the vertebra during PLIF/TLIF surgery, the traditional method is to remove the spinous process and the lamina. The spinous process is the bony projection that comes off the back of each vertebra—they form the bumps you feel when you run your hand down your spine. The lamina is the part of the vertebra that covers the spinal cord—it forms a sort of roof over it. The ligaments and muscles of the spine are attached to the spinous process. Traditionally, to treat serious stenosis in the spine, the spinous process and lamina are simply removed. That opens up the space and decompresses the nerves. Minimally invasive surgery can often be done without removing all of the lamina. We remove just enough of it to decompress the nerves and help with your symptoms.

If you think of the spine as the mast of a sailboat, however, you can see how that approach can cause further problems down the line. The muscles and ligaments of the spine are like the stays that hold the mast vertical and keep it stable. If you take away one of those stays, the mast isn't supported as well and can sway more in the breeze. Similarly, the vertebrae above and below the vertebra that has the surgery can start to wear out because they have less support.

To make the posterior decompression less damaging, I can keep the ligaments intact between the spinous process of the vertebrae above and below. I do this by removing just one side of the lamina and working underneath it to reach the openings on both sides for the nerves and enlarge them to decompress the nerves.

CERVICAL SURGERY

The seven cervical (neck) vertebrae support your head and allow head movements such as nodding, driving, reading, laughing, and eating. When these vertebrae are damaged, they can be very painful and limit your range of head motion severely. Activities such as driving can become difficult. Minimally invasive procedures to repair cervical discs can help relieve the pain and restore range of motion.

ACDF

Fusion surgery is often needed to deal with disc problems in the neck. The ACDF (anterior cervical discectomy and fusion) procedure is similar to the ALIF procedure. I make a small transverse (horizontal) incision in the front of the neck. I try to place it into a natural skin crease so the scar won't be too visible later on; also, that's the way the nerves are aligned in the skin, so I cut through fewer of them. I use my finger to split the short, vertical muscles found in the neck. I very carefully move the trachea, the esophagus, and the blood vessels aside to get to the spine. Once I've made a window and can see the spine, I follow the same procedure as for an ALIF or any other disc surgery to remove the disc, spread the bones apart, and enlarge the nerve openings. I can use an artificial disc in the neck to replace the natural disc. If the patient has extensive arthritis in the area, however, I can't do an artificial disc. I do a fusion with a bone cage instead and also realign the spine because arthritis makes it very crooked. If I need to remove a lot of bone to take the pressure off the nerves, I also do an anterior partial corpectomy through the same incision. I usually have to finish the procedure by putting on a plate in front to stabilize the joint while it heals.

For some patients, an artificial disc is a great option after decompressing the nerves of the neck. An artificial disc can restore a good range of motion while taking pressure off the adjacent discs in the neck. The hope is that this will help the other discs wear out more slowly. Artificial discs also help you heal faster after surgery. Not everyone is a candidate for the artificial disc, but for the right person, it's a great choice.

ARTIFICIAL DISCS

For patients with disc problems in the cervical or lumbar vertebrae, we can replace the damaged disc with an artificial disc made of titanium or other materials instead of fusing the two vertebrae. That lets the patient have a lot more range of motion and flexibility after the surgery. Having more motion at the disc level with an artificial disc can help share the load on the adjacent vertebrae and take pressure off the remaining discs above and below in the spine. That helps protect the other discs and decrease the chance that they'll wear out in the future.

Artificial discs are most suitable for people who have minimal arthritis or minimal damage or disease of the spine. Someone with a lot of arthritic damage, or osteoporosis, or a serious misalignment or deformity of the spine isn't a good candidate. Neither is someone who puts a lot of stress and strain on their neck, like a fighter pilot or professional hockey player. Even in good candidates, pain might continue after the surgery if there are also problems with structures in the back of the neck, such as muscles or the facet joints.

If you are a good candidate—and a lot of people are—the artificial disc is much better than having fusion surgery because it allows you to have continued motion and can protect your other discs as well. Most people have a very quick recovery and get back to their active lifestyle with a big improvement in pain and range of motion.

One potential downside to the artificial disc is that down the road, it can wear out, just like anything else that has motion. It may need to be replaced or revised. The ones we have are lasting a long time and doing very well. Artificial discs are approved in the U.S. only for the cervical and lower lumbar areas. I use them mostly for patients with cervical issues because restoring range of motion to the head and neck makes a big difference. The impact is less in the lower back.

DOWNSIDES TO DISC SURGERY

Every surgery has risks. In spine surgery, you have the standard surgical risks of infection, bleeding, and blood clots. Some risks specific to spine surgery include:

- Nonunion (pseudarthrosis). Nonunion happens when a fusion doesn't heal as expected. Most cases of nonunion occur in people who smoke, are very obese, have diabetes, or have multilevel fusion surgery. If the nonunion causes symptoms, a second surgery may be needed.
- Instrumentation problems. To stabilize the spine as you heal, we put in metal screws, rods, plates, and other devices. After the bone has healed, the instrumentation isn't needed any longer. We simply leave it in place, but sometimes it causes discomfort or breaks. A second operation may be needed to remove it.
- Bone cage problems. The bone cage we use in fusion surgery is held in place by the vertebrae and the instrumentation, but sometimes it can move out place during the early stages of healing. A second surgery may be needed to replace it.
- Damage to the spinal cord or nerves causing pain, weakness, and even paralysis. This complication is rare.

SCOLIOSIS

Fifty years ago, when older people got degenerative scoliosis (too much curve to one side in the spine), we didn't have the tools or hardware we do today. Instead, we would put people into body casts to try to realign the spine. When that didn't work, we would do big surgery on the spine. We'd open up the back, move all the muscles around and do bone grafts hoping they would heal, then sew you up and put you into a body cast for months.

Then the Harrington rod was invented. This was a big, long rod with hooks on each end that we would use to straighten out the curve and then do the fusion. That worked better, but over time, the curve often got too flat, which caused more pain and disability and often needed more surgery.

Today, our techniques and our tools are so much better. We can straighten out the vertebrae by putting screws into each of the vertebral bodies and then use rods and hooks to fix the excess curvature and restore a natural curve instead.

For patients with severe scoliosis, we still need to straighten the curve with open surgery. Bigger surgery is probably better in these cases, even with the risk of needing a transfusion and being in the hospital for a few more days. Open surgery today takes advantage of minimally invasive techniques to protect the nerves and the muscles, decrease bleeding, and improve healing so the risks are reduced and the recovery is faster. A year down the road, these patients do much better. One of my recent scoliosis patients, a college student, had an incision on her back that was almost two feet long. She came in to see me for a follow-up visit two weeks after the surgery wearing a backless dress. She was off pain meds and proud of her skinny scar, because now she was standing tall.

Even with open scoliosis surgery, however, we now use some of the principles of smaller surgery to get better fusion and better healing. For less severe cases, we can now use some techniques that allow a smaller surgery with a faster recovery time. If you've got a curve in the lumbar spine below the ribs but above the pelvis, we can sometimes do the surgery using minimally invasive techniques, without having to open up all the muscles in the back. Instead, we can do two or three disc levels from the front. Using a modified XLIF or OLIF procedure, I can take out the discs and use shims or bone cages to realign the spine and fuse it in place. The incision is much smaller and doesn't cut through muscles. We can get remarkable improvement in the curve. The goal is to help the patient be able to balance their head over their pelvis, instead of being tilted off to one side. Even if we can't get the back completely straight, we can improve the balance and get the arthritic parts stabilized and causing less pain and numbness by taking pressure off the nerves, directly or indirectly.

In fact, the front approach to scoliosis is so effective that a few spine centers are now using a similar approach for kids with scoliosis. For some of these kids, we can fuse just three or four vertebrae in the middle back instead of using a rod to realign and fuse more of the spine. It's still too early to say, but for some of these teens we might be able to give them smaller surgery and more flexibility in the spine afterward. Minimally invasive scoliosis surgery for the right curves has a lot of potential. It would be great if we could do this because the big surgery we do now involves fusion at multiple levels and leaves the spine stiff.

Recognizing and treating scoliosis early is important, even if it requires bigger surgery. Not only does early surgery help with the deformity, it helps protect the function of the lungs, the heart, and other organs. A large curve in the spine compresses organs and decreases their function. By restoring the normal curve or stopping the progression, we can help decrease the pain and decrease the deformity. We can also improve posture. Most importantly, we can improve or at least protect the lung function and heart function.

BERTOLOTTI'S SYNDROME

I wrote an article more than fifteen years ago about Bertolotti's syndrome that still gets people to come see me in Virginia from all over the country. I love to diagnose this rare back problem because it's often missed as a cause of lower back pain. The pain is often mistaken for pain from the sacroiliac joint, so it doesn't get treated correctly.

Bertolotti's syndrome is a congenital problem. When the spine is in the developmental stage before birth, the separate vertebrae in the sacral (pelvic) region fuse together to form one bone called the sacrum. In the lumbar spine, or low back, the lumbar vertebrae develop as separate segments with their own discs, transverse processes, and spinous processes. That allows the lumbar spine to move and gives us flexibility. Sometimes, however, during development, the lowest vertebra in the back, the L5 lumbar vertebra, can't quite decide to be part of the sacrum or not. It doesn't develop normally. The transverse process is often enlarged, but it doesn't fuse with the sacrum. Instead, it forms a transitional vertebra, a sort of fake joint between the vertebra and the sacrum. Most of the time, this doesn't cause any problems, but if the fake joint gets inflamed, it causes low back pain that's very similar to sacroiliac pain or even lumbar facet pain.

If the joint does cause pain, the traditional treatment is to fuse the whole level together so it doesn't move anymore. That doesn't make sense to me—it really limits movement. I've had great success using minimally invasive spine surgery to reshape the enlarged transverse process and make it smaller, the way it should be.

SACROILIAC DYSFUNCTION

The sacroiliac (SI) joint is the strong weight-bearing joint in the pelvis that connects the sacrum and the pelvis. These joints move together as a single unit and provide additional shock absorption for the spine. For a long time, we thought the joint was so rigid that it couldn't move, so it couldn't become unstable. That turns out not to be true. The sacroiliac is no different from any other joint in the body—it can become just as dysfunctional. And when SI joint dysfunction is severe, the pain is felt in the hip, groin, buttocks, and even down the back of the thigh. Back when we believed that the SI joint couldn't be the source of that sort of pain, we often misdiagnosed the pain as coming from degenerative hip disease, hip bursitis, lumbar disc herniation, or pinched nerves.

Fortunately, we now recognize that the SI joint is a potential source of low back pain. In fact, up to 25 percent of patients at spine clinics have been found to have significant pain contribution from the hip or SI joint. Even more fortunately, we now have good treatment options for sacroiliac joint dysfunction. Most patients can be treated nonoperatively through anti-inflammatory medications, physical therapy, or SI joint injections.

Some patients will need surgical treatment to stabilize and fuse the joint. We used to do a complicated procedure that involved removing a piece of bone from the ilium over the sacroiliac joint to expose the cartilage. The cartilage was trimmed, the bone was put back into place, and the joint was stabilized with plates and screws. The patient then had to keep weight off that side by using crutches for three months.

Another way to stabilize the joint was to place hollow screws across the joint. This usually works pretty well. Sometimes these screws loosen and stop stabilizing the joint, and the pain can return. However, for most people, the pain improvement is long-lasting once the joint is stabilized.

I've been doing SI stabilizations and fusions with minimally invasive surgery for more than twenty years. I currently use virtual reality and computer-assisted imaging with these surgeries. Someday fairly soon, we'll be able to do this procedure robotically.

POST-LAMINECTOMY SYNDROME

Although many people get better from having back surgery, some people still have continued pain. These people are often labeled as having post-laminectomy syndrome, also called failed back syndrome. They're often told that everything surgically possible has already been done, and they have to just live with pain.

I don't think that's true for many patients. These people don't have to be in pain for the rest of their lives. I've found that often there's something else wrong in the back that can be treated. It's possible their previous surgery may not have completely fused, or they might be feeling the screws or other hardware that was put into place, or maybe another disc has worn out. I feel it is very important to reevaluate anyone who's still in pain after surgery to see if anything else can be done.

A lot of people with post-laminectomy syndrome end up being treated by pain management doctors. I recommend that they be evaluated every six or twelve months by a spine surgeon just to see if any other options are available. A team approach is the best way to help people with continued pain. The team should include a surgeon along with the other doctors and therapists. No more surgery might be indicated—back pain is just what they have, and we need to help them cope with it. But in my experience, many people have been mislabeled with post-laminectomy syndrome. One more shot at surgery might help them. And if we can improve the pain even somewhat, that makes you feel better and makes the job of pain management easier.

My favorite type of patient is someone who's had a minimally invasive TLIF procedure but is still hurting. Maybe they didn't heal right. I love seeing those people, because most of the time, I can find a way to help them. They finally feel better physically. They also feel better psychologically, because they've been told that they were just stuck with a failed back surgery and would have to live with the pain. I'm their last hope, and it's incredibly gratifying to help them.

SOLVING THE PROBLEM

Spine surgeons used to say, half-jokingly, that once you operate on a patient, you have a customer for life because their spine is going to keep wearing out. Whatever it is in your body that has already let part of your spine wear out doesn't necessarily stop with the surgery. Realistically, other parts are going to wear out as well. So, you might fix something now, but then something else might need to be fixed later on. You could end up having several back surgeries over the years, fixing something different each time.

Fortunately, because of minimally invasive surgery, additional surgery isn't the problem it used to be. When we do minimally invasive surgery, we do less damage and create less scar tissue, so the muscles and ligaments and tendons aren't so disrupted. That means the vertebrae above and below are more protected and have less chance of wearing out years later. Similarly, when we do minimally invasive scoliosis surgery, we get your spine back to a better curve and let you balance your head above your pelvis again. That means there's less focal stress on the spine for other areas to wear out. If you do need additional surgery down the road, it's easier because you have less scarring and other damage from the previous operation.

DO IT NOW

I've gone through all the various types of common minimally invasive spine surgeries for back pain so that you can have a good idea of what each procedure involves. Now that you understand what's involved, you're much closer to making a good, informed decision with your surgeon.

If you truly need surgery, try not to delay. I had a patient recently who needed surgery for a simple disc herniation. The insurance company took more than a year to approve it. When we delay, the chances of a good result go down. In the case of my patient, he didn't heal well and we needed to do another surgery. You can imagine, the longer the nerve is irritated, the more damage can occur. Just like having a pebble in your shoe, it irritates, but if you get the pebble out early, you are fine. However, if you leave it in for months, you may get sores and ulcers that may not heal well. The same analogy can work when treating other problems, like disc herniations. The insurance companies try to keep from having to pay for the surgery by delaying it. Then, when the surgery doesn't work as well because of the delay, they use that as a reason to say back surgery doesn't work at all.

You have the power to affect your diagnosis, and surgery may not be the answer. But it is important to get a good diagnosis. With this diagnosis, we can discuss the probabilities and results of different treatments. Often, it is appropriate to do nonoperative treatment. Other times, surgery is more "conservative." It is important to be a participant in your health. Be involved and do the work needed to learn and get better.

Conclusion

You, the patient, have much within your own power to affect your diagnosis. Most back pain is caused by lifestyle: being overweight, eating an inflammatory diet, smoking, using too much alcohol, and being sedentary. But lifestyle can be modified—and so can your back pain.

If you optimize your health, you can optimize the chances that whatever is causing your back pain can be treated without surgery just by helping your body heal itself naturally. By exercising and being active, you can maintain your flexibility and strength and keep good heart and lung function. Your exercise can be as simple as walking and aiming for 10,000 steps a day. If you add in some stretching, yoga exercises, and maybe even some resistance training with weights, so much the better.

You also have it in your power to get your movement back.

If your doctor recommends physical therapy for your back pain, do it. Work with your PT and do your home exercises to build up your muscles and get the flexibility back in your ligaments.

By having good nutrition with plenty of good protein and fats and avoiding sugar and bad carbohydrates, you can maintain or achieve normal body weight. By avoiding poor-quality foods, you avoid the inflammation that contributes to back pain and slows its healing. Add in supplements of vitamin C, vitamin D, and fish oil to help keep inflammation to a minimum.

By staying active and engaged in your community, you stay healthier in general. You'll be physically and mentally stronger. You'll be more resilient and able to get through a bout of back pain without it turning into a chronic problem that leads to surgery.

Minimally invasive surgery doesn't magically cure you, though it can make you feel much better. More importantly, the surgery helps you get back to physical therapy and a regular exercise program. When you do rehab and move, you stimulate your body to heal itself and regain its strength. If you just sit back after the surgery and don't move, the surgery won't be very helpful in the end. You'll also be risking getting pneumonia, blood clots, and osteoporosis if you don't move.

HOPE FOR FAILED BACK SURGERY

Many of my new patients have had previous back surgery elsewhere that failed. They're still in pain, or they're in pain again, and they've been told surgery isn't an option anymore. They're told, wrongly, that nothing more can be done.

In very few cases, that's true. But for most victims of failed back surgery, another surgery or intervention is an option. The original surgery may not have been thorough enough, or the patient didn't heal well, or maybe the surgery didn't get to the real source of the problem.

Here's what I often see: The patient has stenosis in the lower back. The surgeon operates to take the pressure off the nerve, but doesn't go on to stabilize that section of the spine. The patient feels better for a while, but because the spine is still moving, eventually the symptoms come back. The surgeon then says, "You already had surgery and it failed, so I can't operate again. Just take these dangerous pain medications for the rest of your life instead." You're considered a failed patient, but actually, your surgery was successful—it's just that it was incomplete. The benefits didn't last.

I often see cases where the patient is in pain again because the original surgeon didn't do enough of a discectomy to repair the disc space, or the spine didn't fuse well. I can help by basically completing the job the original surgeon started. The surgery is more difficult because of the previous work, and there's still a chance it will fail, but I think it's worthwhile to give you a good shot at getting back to a more acceptable quality of life.

Surgery is often thought of as an aggressive treatment, as opposed to conservative treatments, meaning nonoperative treatments. In surgery, conservative means doing the least aggressive operation you can consistent with solving the problem and helping the patient feel better. If you've got a nail in your foot, the most conservative thing you can do is surgery to take it out. If you've got a pinched nerve in your back due to a big herniation and your foot and leg are getting weaker and weaker as a result, it doesn't make sense to just try a little nonoperative therapy to see if it gets better. It won't. You've got a herniated disc in your back; you need the pressure taken off your nerve. The best treatment that will have a good short-term and long-term outcome should be the most conservative treatment, and often that's surgery.

EDUCATE YOURSELF

I wrote this book because I want you to educate yourself about your health, your back pain, and your options. I want you to come to me ready to advocate for yourself based on solid knowledge. I want to diagnose your problem and recommend a treatment and have you say, "From what I already know and what you've told me, that makes sense. Let's do it." What I don't want you to say is, "You're the doctor, I'll just do whatever you say." I want you to go into surgery with realistic expectations about what I can do and what you have to do to make your surgery a success.

I can do a lot, but I can't make you perfect again, and I can't promise you'll be a hundred percent pain-free after the surgery. I can tell you that eight out of ten people who have spine surgery for back pain tell me their pain is cut at least in half, and many are pain-free. If that makes sense for you, if your life would be truly improved with your pain reduced by half from what it is now, then we can talk.

FINAL THOUGHTS

Most people with back problems don't need surgery. To get better, you need to get a good, accurate diagnosis and follow that up with directed treatment, either nonoperative or surgical, for the best chance of having the best results. In many cases, if surgery is needed, the best results will be from minimally invasive surgery that gets you back to the best active life you can have.

If you're having back pain that nothing else is helping, surgery may be right for you. If you've had a failed back surgery, there's hope—more surgery may still be right for you. I'd like to help. To arrange a consultation, please call my office at (703) 936-9474. Or visit my website www.HaszMD.com. Other contact methods and social media can be found on the website.

About the Author

A nationally recognized spinal specialist, MICHAEL HASZ, MD, FACS, is a spinal surgeon at the Hasz Spine Institute in Reston, Virginia, and was listed among the country's top 1 percent of physicians in his specialty by *US News & World Report*. A former major in the US Air Force, Dr. Hasz was chairman of the department of orthopedic surgery and director of spinal surgery at the Andrews Air Force Base / Malcolm Grow Medical Clinics and Surgery Center. He currently holds an appointment as clinical instructor of orthopedic surgery and assistant professor of surgery at the Uniformed Services University of the Health Sciences in Bethesda, Maryland.

Made in the USA
Coppell, TX
10 November 2026

11835574R00111